Yalanda R.

10/27/83

The Development of
Auditory Behavior

The Development of Auditory Behavior

Edited by

Sanford E. Gerber

Speech and Hearing Center
University of California
Santa Barbara, California

George T. Mencher

School of Human Communication Disorders
Dalhousie University
Nova Scotia Hearing and Speech Clinic
Halifax, Nova Scotia
Canada

Grune & Stratton
A Subsidiary of Harcourt Brace Jovanovich, Publishers

New York   London
Paris   San Diego   San Francisco   São Paulo
Sydney   Tokyo   Toronto

Grune & Stratton, Inc.
111 Fifth Avenue
New York, New York 10003

Distributed in the United Kingdom by
Academic Press Inc. (London) Ltd.
24/28 Oval Road, London NW 1

Library of Congress Catalog Number 83-48111
International Standard Book Number 0-8089-1598-3
Printed in the United States of America

Contents

III Linguistic Development

IV Conclusions

Foreword

The volume that follows is the fruit of a conference on the development of auditory behavior. Often, conference participants have to be exhorted of the importance of their mission. It was refreshing not to have to convince anyone in this small and distinguished group of the importance of better understanding of the development of auditory behavior and of deriving more perceptive views of abnormal auditory behavior, especially in infants.

On the other hand, the need for zeal satisfied, how could this conference be justified? The participants should already have known how auditory behavior develops. They have watched the development in their own and other children. Furthermore, each participant has researched one or several facets of auditory behavior. Why, then, was it deemed valuable to convene a panel of experts on the topic? What could the conference, and the present book, contribute that was not already known?

In its narrowest sense, auditory behavior connotes overt responses to acoustic signals. However, even those persons whose main concern is overt behavioral response to sound realize that overt behavior is an end product. This result does not tell us why or how the behavior evolved to its present state, and it may not be a sufficient predictor of future auditory behavior, normal or abnormal.

To appreciate the implications of overt auditory behavior, one should have some understanding of the genetic background and of the embryologic development of the auditory mechanism. One should have some knowledge of the anatomic and physiologic substrate of audition. Understanding the physical signals and their psychophysical processing is also essential. Knowledge of the psychosocial milieu in which auditory behavior develops is also important to the cognition of auditory behavior in infants.

These are only samples from the catalog of facets of auditory behavior and its development. Much can be gained from concentrated study of any one of these elements. Can greater advancement be made, however, by combining observations from studies of two or more facets? Can the combined observations be integrated into a better or fuller view of auditory behavior? Can something be learned from the integration of the pieces to help us better comprehend the abnormalities of auditory behavior, especially in infants? Finally, can greater understanding of abnormalities of development lead to improved means of remediating disordered auditory behavior?

The above questions helped to define the purpose of the recent conference. The participants had no illusions that they could conquer even a restricted corner of the world in one short conference. Nevertheless, they hoped and expected to progress a significant step in the direction toward better understanding of the development of auditory behavior, of abnormalities in its development, and of ways to improve faulty auditory behavior. The contents of this book reflect at least a modest fulfillment of the hopes of the conference organizers and participants.

Any conference of this nature serves additional useful purposes: the identification of unanswered questions and unresolved problems, and the direction of thought to new avenues of clinical and laboratory observation and research. These queries indeed may be some of the more valuable aspects of the conference proceedings.

Finally, another valuable outcome of the conference was the profitable influence of the serious and objective criticism of the participants on one another. This effect may be difficult to sense in the printed pages; nevertheless, it was clearly felt by the participants. They knew that their own work would benefit from the knowledgeable criticisms, suggestions, and information received at the conference. They will feel even more rewarded if their words which follow will have a similar salutory impact on the readers.

Robert Goldstein

Preface

Ever since 1974, we have had the good fortune to co-chair a series of conferences on the hearing impaired infant. In reviewing these published volumes, we recognized that there is no such volume on the normal infant, particularly one promoting the idea that an understanding of the hearing impaired infant must be derived from the study of normal auditory behavior. A couple of years ago, we reported this observation to the National Foundation, March of Dimes, soliciting their support to assemble the group of scholars represented herein. We are indebted to them for that support.

Our aim in assembling these contributions was to note the anatomical and physiological bases of auditory development, the acoustic and psychoacoustic bases of auditory development, and the linguistic and psycholinguistic bases of auditory development. In our opinion, this is an extraordinary volume. The contributions of anatomists, audiologists, and linguists addressed to this single issue is a novel and pivotal publishing event. We are indebted to the March of Dimes for supporting it originally and continue to appreciate the willingness of Grune & Stratton to publish our works.

We are also especially indebted to three people who have worked very hard to assemble this volume for publication. Joyce Gauvain made most of the arrangements for the original conference, did most of the bibliographic work, and cleaned up the typing of all the contributors. She was aided by Holly Haggerty who did the bibliographies and some of the indexes. Jane Mahneke did the final typing of the entire manuscript essentially error-free; that is a significant accomplishment. These people made it possible for us to publish and for you to read what we believe to be significant materials.

Sanford E. Gerber
George T. Mencher

Contributors

Donald G. Doehring, Ph.D.
School of Human Communication Disorders
McGill University, Montreal, Quebec, Canada

Sanford E. Gerber, Ph.D.
Speech and Hearing Center
University of California, Santa Barbara, California

Kurt Hecox, M.D., Ph.D.
Department of Neurology
Waisman Center on Mental Retardation and Human Development
University of Wisconsin, Madison, Wisconsin

Ivan Hunter-Duvar, Ph.D.
Department of Otolaryngology
University of Toronto, Toronto, Ontario, Canada

Roberta L. Klatzky, Ph.D.
Department of Psychology
University of California, Santa Barbara, California

Patrica K. Kuhl, Ph.D.
Department of Speech and Hearing Sciences
Child Development and Mental Retardation Center
University of Washington, Seattle, Washington

George T. Mencher, Ph.D.
School of Human Communication Disorders
Dalhousie University, Nova Scotia Hearing and Speech Clinic
Halifax, Nova Scotia, Canada

Lenore S. Mencher
Hearing Screening Program
Nova Scotia Hearing and Speech Clinic
Halifax, Nova Scotia, Canada

Maurice I. Mendel, Ph.D.
Speech and Hearing Center
University of California, Santa Barbara, California

D. Kimbrough Oller, Ph.D.
Department of Pediatrics and Psychology
Mailman Center for Child Development
University of Miami, Miami, Florida

Agnes H. Ling Phillips, Ph.D.
Montreal Oral School for the Deaf, Montreal, Quebec, Canada

Carol A. Prutting, Ph.D.
Speech and Hearing Center
University of California, Santa Barbara, California

Robert J. Ruben, M.D.
Department of Otorhinolaryngology
Albert Einstein College of Medicine
Yeshiva University, Bronx, New York

Bruce A. Schneider, Ph.D.
Center for Research in Human Development
Erindale College, University of Toronto
Mississauga, Ontario, Canada

Sandra E. Trehub, Ph.D.
Center for Research in Human Development
Erindale College, University of Toronto
Mississauga, Ontario, Canada

Thomas R. Van De Water, Ph.D.
Laboratory of Developmental Otobiology
Department of Otorhinolaryngology
Albert Einstein College of Medicine
Yeshiva University, Bronx, New York

Wesley R. Wilson, Ph.D.
Department of Speech and Hearing Sciences
Child Development and Mental Retardation Center
University of Washington, Seattle, Washington

Part I

Biological Development

RECENT ADVANCES IN THE DEVELOPMENTAL
BIOLOGY OF THE INNER EAR

Robert J. Ruben
Thomas R. Van De Water
Albert Einstein College of Medicine of Yeshiva University

INTRODUCTION

The incidence and effects of congenital sensory-neural
deafness are well known. The causes of congenital deafness
are thought to be approximately 50% genetic and 50% acquired
(Fraser, 1976). Hearing losses which occur during postnatal
life of an individual have also been categorized as being
either of genetic or acquired origin. The proportions of
these postnatal hearing losses which are genetic are unknown.
It is estimated that the prevalence of genetic disease as
the etiological factor of hearing loss in the elderly is
approximately 50% (Ruben and Kruger, in preparation). Genetic
disease, although becoming manifest in later life, is fundamentally congenital. A broader view of "congenital" diseases
of the inner ear would be to include all etiologies which
occur in utero and result in deficits either pre or postpartum. With these considerations, it is evident that much
of sensory-neural hearing loss affecting the population is
fundamentally congenital in origin.

Diseases are controlled in three ways: prevention, cure,
and care. During the past decade, there have been significant advances taken in the area of prevention of acquired,
congenital, and postpartum hearing loss. There has been the
advent of Rubella vaccine, Rh immunization, the identification
of ototoxic substances, and programs to control against excessive noise exposure. There are, at present, no preventive
or cure interventions for sensory-neural hearing loss of genetic origin with the exception of genetic counselling. The
only efficacious interventions which are available for these
diseases are those of care. It is the mission of otology to
be able to prevent or cure these genetic sensory-neural
hearing losses. In order that this may be accomplished,
there must be an acquisition of knowledge of the embryologic

mechanisms which control the expression of normal inner ear
development and the mechanisms by which mutated genes disrupt
these developmental mechanisms and cause hearing loss. As
all of these diseases are primarily congenital in nature, then
the study of prenatal development of the inner ear becomes
mandatory.

The sequence of anatomical events which occurs in the
development of the mammalian inner ear has been well known
since the end of the 19th century and the beginning of the
20th century (Held, 1909; Retzius, 1884). The time at which
the auditory receptor cells of mammalian inner ear were
formed (i.e., underwent their terminal mitotic division) was
reported by Ruben (1967). These studies from the mouse ear,
in a general way, can be applied to what occurs in man. Ex-
trapolating from the mouse data, it would appear that the
cells which compose Corti's organ in man probably undergo
their terminal mitoses before the end of the second month of
gestation, i.e., at the juncture of the end of the embryonic
period and the beginning of the fetal period. This information suggests that many of the abnormalities seen in both
acquired and genetic congenital sensory-neural hearing losses
may occur in the embryonic period, i.e., during the early
placode to otocyst stage of inner ear development.

The ability to perform experimental manipulations on
mammalian otocysts in utero is limited. To be able to study
the factors which control the normal and abnormal development of the inner ear, a reproducable and reliable organ
culture technique was developed by Van De Water and Ruben
(1971, 1973). The ability to grow the mammalian inner ear in
organ culture in our laboratory has permitted a systematic
study of the cellular factors, and currently, to begin to
examine the biochemical mechanisms which control the expression of normal inner ear development. The following text
discusses some of our more recent observations concerning
embryonic mechanisms which act to guide normal development
of the inner ear and manipulations of these developmental
mechanisms that result in formation of an abnormal inner ear.

MORPHOLOGY

As part of a systematic ultrastructural study of the
early stages of embryonic development of the inner ear, observations were made concerning the relationships of the otic
placode to the adjacent rhombencephalon and surrounding periotic mesenchyme (see Figs. 1-1 and 1-2). No cellular contacts

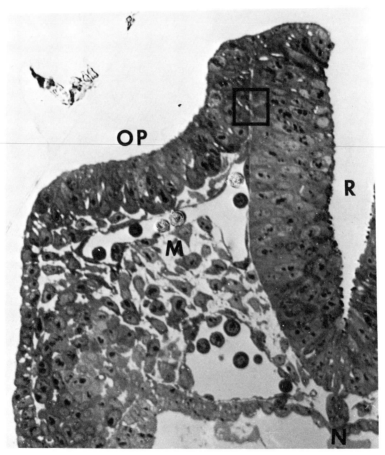

Figure 1-1. A cross section of an otic placode and the
adjacent rhombencephalon. The area of closest apposition
between neuroepithelial cells of the otic placode and rhombencephalon is enclosed in a box (X500). (See figure legends
for all figures at the end of the chapter).

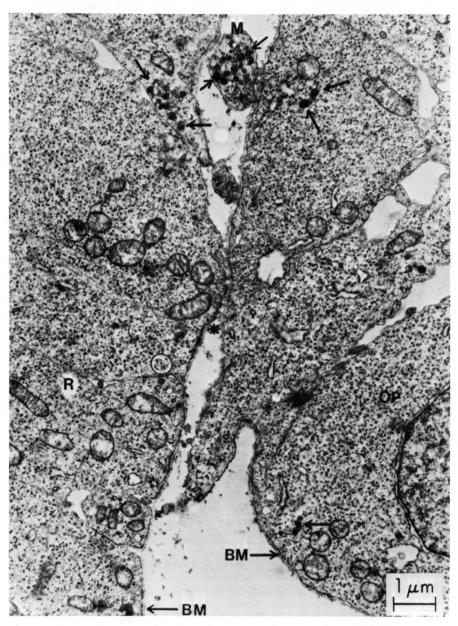

Figure 1-2. A transmission electron micrograph of the area of
closest cellular apposition between neuroepithelial cells of
the otic placode and rhombencephalon. Note that the integrity
of the basement membranes is not lost in these areas and that
sparse, or no, extracellular matrix is present.

between placodal and rhombencephalic tissue were detected when
the areas of closest apposition of these two tissues were
serially sectioned and ultrastructurally examined. This ultrastructural analysis showed that these two tissue types were
always seen to be separated by their basement membranes. This
observation suggests that brain tissue does not exert its
earliest inductive influence via membrane to membrane contact
with the otic anlagen.

    Ultrastructural studies of the relationship of the otic
cup, the adjacent rhombencephalon, and its surrounding mesenchyme (Fig. 1-3) show that there are no areas of cellular
contact between the cells of the otic cup and those of the
rhombencephalon (Fig. 1-4). Cellular processes of the surrounding periotic mesenchyme are shown to penetrate the basement membranes of both the otic anlagen and the adjacent
rhombencephalon (Fig. 1-5). This suggests that one of the
embryonic mechanisms in inner ear development may be that one
of the ways the rhombencephalon exerts its early inductive
control on development of the inner ear is via the intervening
periotic mesenchyme cells. These observations of the differences in the cellular relationships between the otic placode
and its neighboring rhombencephalon and periotic mesenchyme
suggest the hypothesis that the early development of the inner
ear may be more directly controlled by periotic mesenchyme
than by the rhombencephalon. This hypothesis is intuitively
formed based upon our ultrastructural observations and needs
further experimental testing for validation.

NORMAL GENE EXPRESSION

    Two organ culture studies of gene expression of the
normal development of the inner ear are of interest. The first
of these demonstrates that on the 11th and 12th days of gestation the cells which compose the otocyst, although homogeneous,
are already committed to become specific sensory organelles
and cell types of the inner ear (Li et al., 1978). This experiment consisted of surgically dividing an otocyst in half
along one of three different planes of section which resulted
in otic explants composed of medial-lateral, anterior-posterior,
or dorsal-ventral halves. These inner ear segments were explanted to organ culture to allow for further development of
inner ear sensory structures and subsequent analysis of their
histologic development. A summary of the results is represented in Fig. 1-6. The data show that the ventral half of
the otocyst has been pre-programmed to form the cochlear duct
and saccule. Further analysis of the results demonstrates the

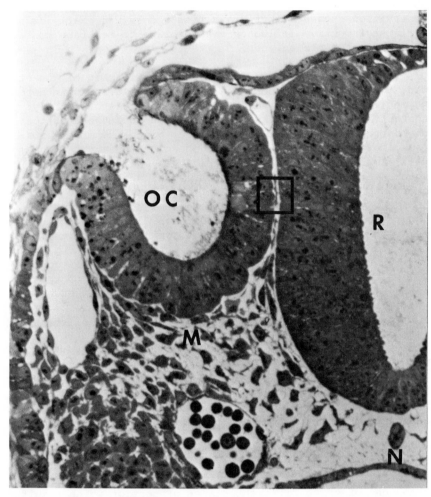

Figure 1-3. A cross section of an otic cup and the adjacent rhombencephalon. The area of closest cellular apposition between neuroepithelial cells of the otic cup and rhombencephalon is enclosed in a box. Note the intervening mesenchymal cell processes (X500).

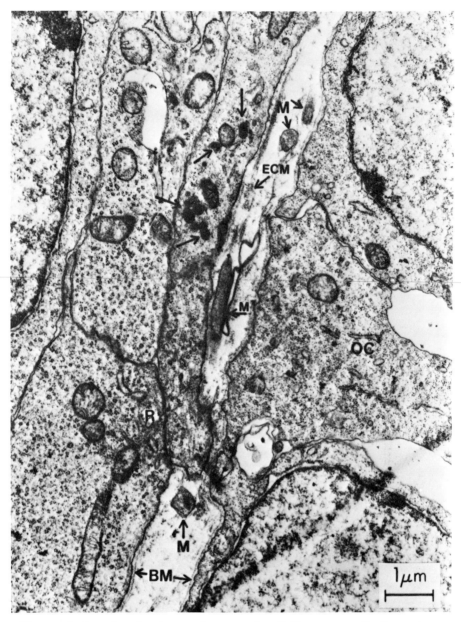

Figure 1-4. An electron micrograph of the area of closest apposition between neuroepithelial cells of the otic cup and rhombencephalon. The integrity of the basement membranes of these closely apposed tissues is intact. Mesenchyme cell processes are frequently seen in the cleft between these tissues and there has been a marked increase in the presence and quantity of extracellular matrix.

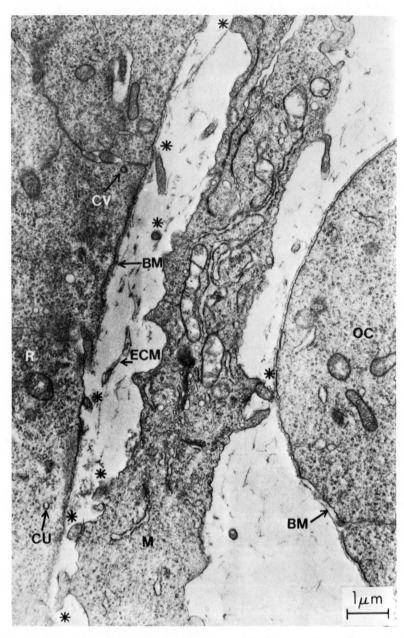

Figure 1-5. An electron micrograph of the cleft between the otic cup and the rhombencephalon. A large process of a cephalic mesenchyme cell is seen making contact with the basement membranes of both the otic cup and rhombencephalon as well as the extracellular matrix found within the cleft.

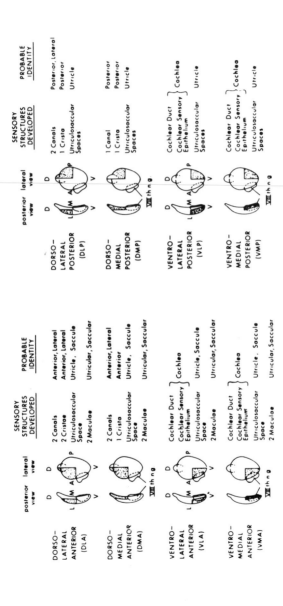

Figure 1-6. Summary chart of the fate mapping of the eight anatomical sectors of the mouse otocyst (reprinted from J. Morph. 157:249-268, 1978 with permission).

11

high specificity of the "homogeneous" cells of the 11 and 12
day otocyst; e.g., the crista and ampulla of the anterior
semicircular duct are derived from the dorso-anterior quadrant
of the otocyst. This experiment reveals that the genetic
mechanisms for expression of differentiation of the various
portions of the inner ear are programmed within the inner
ear anlagen by the 11th day of embryonic life in the mouse
model system. This information, taken as a whole, provides
a fate map of the developing otocyst (see Fig. 1-6) which
becomes a basis for study of what types of manipulations
can be done to effect the normal developmental mechanisms
that would affect both morphologic and cytologic expression
of the labyrinthine development.

A second experimental series of interest concerns the
mechanism by which afferent nerve fibers of the eighth nerve
innervate sensory cells of the inner ear. It has been shown
(Sher, 1971) that afferent dendrites which grow from the
statoacoustic ganglion do not reach the otocyst until the
12th day of gestation. It has also been demonstrated (Van De
Water, 1976) that sensory structures of the inner ear are
able to undergo normal morphogenesis and cytodifferentiation
in organ culture in the absence of any neurotrophic influence
that may be provided by ingrowing afferent nerve fibers. The
next question asked was if neurotrophic interactions occur
between developing sensory hair cells and ingrowing dendrites
of the eighth nerve; and if so, are they specific or general?
The following preliminary study is designed to investigate
the feasibility of applying the "in vitro" system to questions of neurotrophic interactions and neuronal specificity.

This study was performed as follows. Pairs of otocysts
were removed from 12.5 day embryos; from one otocyst, the
statoacoustic ganglion was removed while in the other otocyst, this ganglion was left intact. These pairs of otocysts
were then explanted into organ culture chambers and co-
cultured in an orientation so that the statoacoustic ganglion
of the intact otocyst was adjacent to the excision site of
ganglion removal of the other otocyst (see Fig. 1-7). These
co-cultured inner ear explants were allowed to further
develop for eight days "in vitro", after which they were then
fixed and histologically processed with nerve fiber stains.
Analysis with light microscopic techniques showed that afferent nerve fibers (Fig. 1-8) had grown into the areas of
developing sensory structures within both otocysts. These
preliminary results show that an ingrowth of eighth nerve
neuronal elements into the aganglionic otocysts had occurred

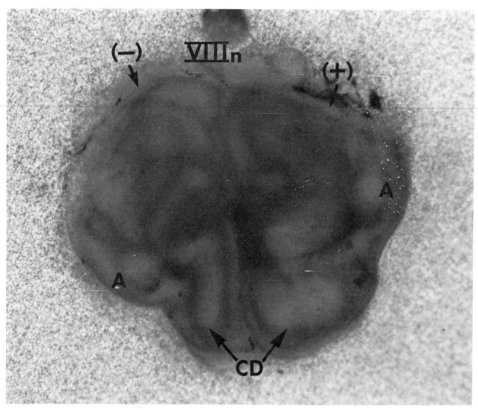

Figure 1-7. Co-cultured 12.5 day otocyst explants, eight days *in vitro*. Right otocyst was explanted with ganglion, left otocyst without ganglion. (X180).

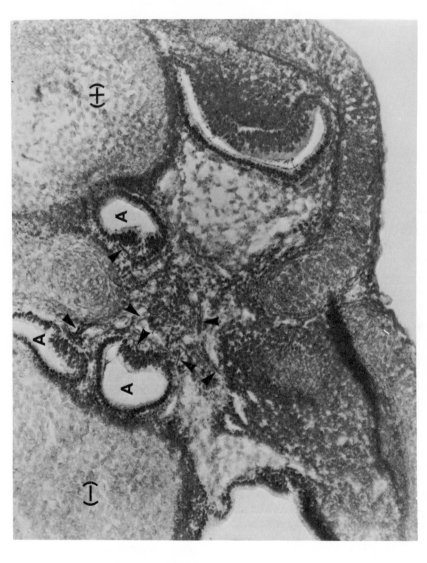

Figure 1-8. Co-cultured 12.5 day otocyst explants, eight days in vitro. A photomicrograph of a histologic cross section through the explants of Figure 1-7 (Bodian stained for neural elements). Nerve fibers (arrowheads) were seen associated with the sensory structures of both explants.

and that these nerve fibers grew preferentially to the sensory structures which were located closest to their source within the co-cultured otocyst explants with intact ganglions. Whether or not there was a decrease in the afferent innervation of the intact otocyst is currently being investigated.

This study shows that some aspects of the neurotrophic interactions that occur during the phase of preliminary outgrowth of neuronal processes from the statoacoustic ganglion towards their target site of the differentiating inner ear sensory structures may be studied in the "in vitro" systems. The results also suggest that those areas of the developing otocyst that are committed to forming sensory receptors may, prior to overt cytodifferentiation, undergo a biochemical differentiation and consequently be active in establishing chemo-attractant fields which may act to direct the ingrowth of neuronal elements from a nearby source to their target sites. Further studies are planned which are designed to further investigate the mechanism of nerve fiber ingrowth into areas of differentiating sensory receptors and the role of this mechanism in neuronal specificity within the developing labyrinth.

FACTORS REGULATING SEQUENTIAL GENE EXPRESSION

The rhombencephalon and periotic mesenchyme which surrounds the otocyst have been identified as two tissues which exert control over the normal development of the inner ear, i.e., normal sequential expression of the genetic messages that orchestrate the development of the inner ear. The study of the rhombencephalic contribution to induction of the inner ear was performed by the study of 9.5, 10, and 10.5 day otocysts under two different conditions using either transfilter tissue interaction techniques or direct tissue contact methods (Figs. 1-9 and 1-10). In the transfilter tissue interaction series, 9.5, 10, and 10.5-day-old mouse otocyst explants were continuously interacted via a 1.0μ average pore diameter (APD) Nuclepore filter membrane with either a plasma clot as a control, or a 12 day rhombencephaic tissue explant held in place with a plasma clot. These explants were cultured for a period of ten days "in vitro" with daily microscopic observations of the cultures. Any advances in morphogenesis were noted and serial micrographs were made of selected explants of the different age groups. The specimens were fixed on the tenth day of "in vitro" development and processed for histology. Histologic quantification of the development of sensory structures was performed by light

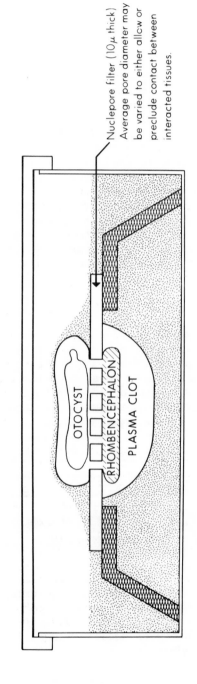

Nuclepore filter (10 μ thick) Average pore diameter may be varied to either allow or preclude contact between interacted tissues.

OTOCYST

RHOMBENCEPHALON

PLASMA CLOT

Figure 1-9. A schematic representation of an in vitro transfilter interaction apparatus.

16

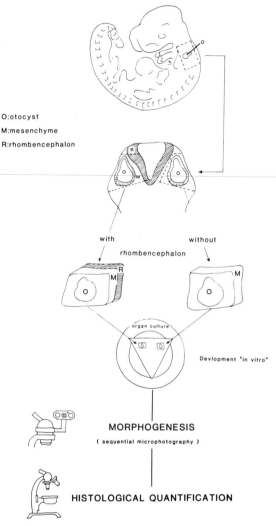

MOUSE EMBRYO (9.5–10–10.5 day)

O:otocyst
M:mesenchyme
R:rhombencephalon

with   without

rhombencephalon

organ culture

Devlopment "in vitro"

MORPHOGENESIS

(sequential microphotography)

HISTOLOGICAL QUANTIFICATION

Figure 1-10. A representation of the experimental design of the direct contact series of otocyst/rhombencephalon induction experiments.

17

microscopic analysis of the sensory structures that had
developed within these otocyst explants. The morphological
results were as follows: at two days of "in vitro" development, no detectable differences could be observed between the
otocyst cultures interacting with rhombencephalon and those
interacting with plasma clots. After four days of "in vitro"
development, the 9.5 and 10-day-old otocyst explants interacted with plasma clots had begun to exhibit degenerative
changes; while otocysts of these same gestational ages interacted with rhombencephalon tissue showed slight advances in
morphogenesis (see Fig. 1-11). After six and eight days in
culture, the plasma clot control cultures of 9.5 and 10-day-
old otocysts had totally degenerated; whereas equivalent
aged otocysts interacted with rhombencephalic tissue showed
definite advances in morphogenesis. The morphogenesis of the
10.5-day-old otocyst explants was similar for both groups
either with or without rhombencephalic tissue in all of the
"in vitro" days mentioned in the above text. The results of
the histologic quantification of sensory structures illustrate that none of the twenty-nine 9.5-day-old otocyst
explants interacted for ten days with plasma clots formed
any sensory structures, and all of those cultured underwent
extensive degenerative changes (see Fig. 1-12). There were
thirty-one 9.5-day-old otocyst explants transfilter interacted with rhombencephalic tissue for ten days, and of these
explants, 87% showed advances in differentiation of the otic
capsule and 64% showed some advanced differentiation of inner
ear sensory structures. In the 10-day otocyst explants,
interacted for ten days with plasma clots, only 13% survived
without degenerative changes and 7% produced differentiation
of an area which contained some sensory hair cells. These
plasma clot controls are compared to the ten day rhombencephalon interacted 10-day otocyst explants, of which all
advanced in morphogenesis and 82% produced advances in differentiation of inner ear sensory structures. The 10.5-day-
old explants of both groups yielded similar results, with the
rhombencephalon transfilter interacted explants showing
slightly more advanced differentiation of sensory structures.
The data indicate that 9.5 and 10-day-old otocysts are
dependent upon the inductive influences of rhombencephalic
tissue for continued development, and that the 10.5-day-old
otocysts explanted in the transfilter series of neural induction did not require interaction with rhombencephalon for
continued development "in vitro", although those explants
that were interacted with rhombencephalon showed quantita-
tively better differentiation of sensory structures (Fig.
1-12).

A second experimental series was done to examine if there is a continuing influence of inductive control exerted by the rhombencephalon (brainstem) on the later stages of morphogenesis and cytodifferentiation of inner ear sensory receptors. This study consisted of 10, 10.5 and 11-day otocyst explants. Within these explants, otic and brainstem tissues were interacted by direct contact with one another and were never separated by an interposed filter membrane. All otocysts were excised with their rhombencephalic tissue intact. The otocysts were explanted as matched pairs from the same embryo, with one otocyst explanted with rhombencephalic tissue intact, whereas the contralateral otocyst underwent additional microsurgery for removal of the attached rhombencephalic tissue. Serial microphotographs and daily microscopic observations revealed that all of the otocyst explants with attached rhombencephalic tissue produced much greater advances in morphogenesis when compared to cultures of their contralateral otocysts that were explanted without rhombencephalic tissue. The morphogenesis of both vestibular and cochlear structures were affected in the 10-day otic explants that lacked rhombencephalon tissue. A comparison between the two types of ten day explants showed that the explants interacting with neural tissue form semi-circular ducts and a hooked cochlear duct. In comparison, the 10-day otic explant alone did not undergo advances in the morphogenesis to form a definable inner ear geometry. The 10.5-day explants did not show as great an effect on the morphogenesis of vestibular structures, but the formation of the cochlear duct was still severely affected by the lack of neural interaction with rhombencephalon (see Fig. 1-13). The effect on the morphogenesis of 11-day specimens was limited specifically to development of the cochlear duct. The otic explants that did not directly interact with rhombencephalon produced cystic outgrowths in comparison to the partially coiled cochlear ducts that developed in the otic explants that included rhombencephalic tissue (see Fig. 1-14). The above descriptive events are based upon observations in over one hundred organ cultured explants and a manuscript detailing these results is in preparation.

EPITHELIAL/MESENCHYMAL TISSUE INTERACTIONS

The microsurgical series consisted of over 250 inner ear explants in which the dependency of normal otic development upon the presence of a critical mass of periotic mesenchyme tissue was assessed. These investigations have shown that the tissue interactions occurring between the surrounding

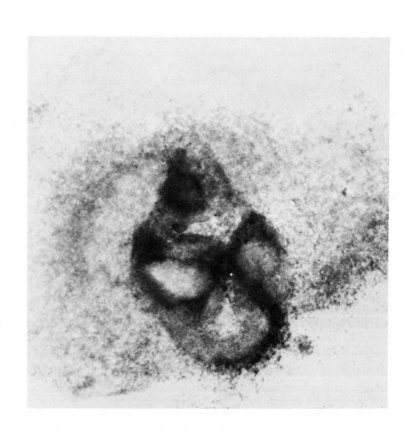

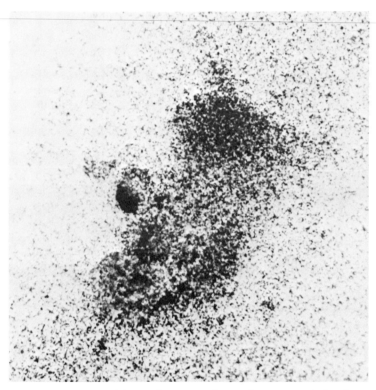

*Figure 1-11. Transfilter interaction of otocyst/rhombenceph-
alon. A matched pair of 9.5 day otocyst interacted with 10
day rhombencephalon (left otocyst) or plasma clots (right
otocyst) for 20 days in vitro. (X100)*

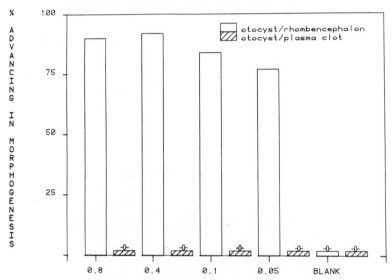

TRANSFILTER INTERACTED INNER EAR*/RHOMBENCEPHALON** EXPLANTS

* 9.5 DAY-OLD OTOCYSTS
** 10 DAY-OLD RHOMBENCEPHALON TISSUE

Figure 1-12. Transfilter interaction histogram. Filter pore diameter below 0.2 microns prohibits cell contact between interacted tissues, but allows free exchange of molecules.

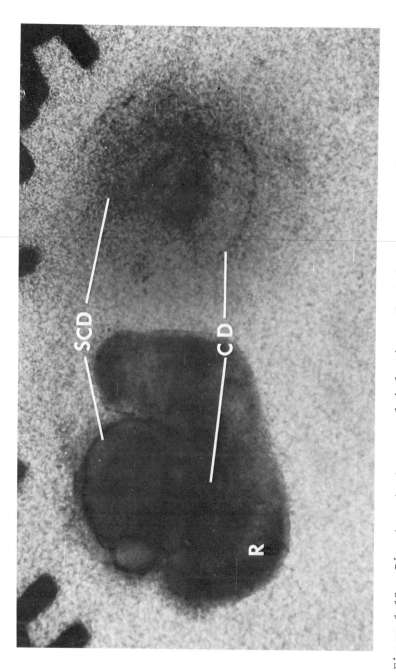

Figure 1-13. Direct contact – neural induction. 10.5 day otocyst explants, 10 days in vitro. Left explant (with rhombencephalon) shows normal otic morphogenesis; right explant (without rhombencephalon) both vestibular and cochlear areas exhibit dysmorphogenesis (X180)

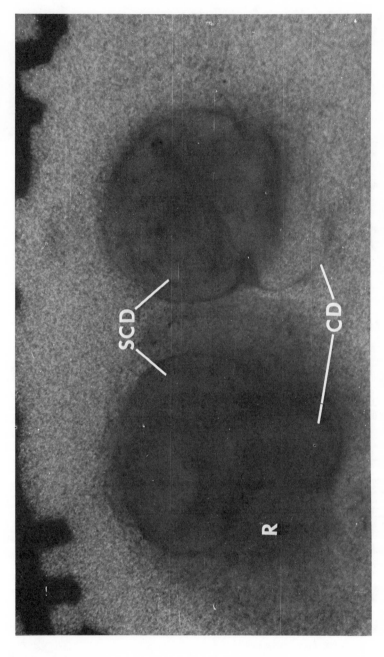

Figure 1-14. Direct contact - neural induction. 11 day otocyst explants, nine days in vitro. Left explant (with rhombencephalon) shows normal otic morphogenesis; right explant (without rhombencephalon) exhibits normal development of vestibular structures and dysmorphogenesis of the cochlear duct.

periotic mesenchyme and the epithelium of the developing
otocyst are critical for the sequential expression of the
genes that code for labyrinthine development. The results
of these studies have revealed a temporal pattern in this
sequential expression of the morphogenesis and cytodifferentiation of the inner ear. In explants of 10.5-day otocysts,
a reduction of mesenchyme volume produces, following a period
of "in vitro" development, only simple flat areas of sensory
cells with no accompanying morphogenesis or cytodifferentiation of any specific sensory receptors. "In vitro" histo-
genesis of vestibular sensory structures in explants of
reduced mesenchyme volume start to occur within specimens
explanted from 11-day embryos. Cytodifferentiation of the
sensory hair cells of auditory sensory areas first occurs in
reduced mesenchyme explants of 11.5-day gestation embryos.
Thus, the tissue interactions occurring between the otocyst
and its surrounding periotic mesenchyme appear to play a vital
role in the sequential expression of the developmental program
of the membranous labyrinth occurring within the epithelial
cells of the otocyst. When these epithelio-mesenchymal tissue
interactions are prevented or modified, a reproducible malformation of the inner ear occurs which is directly related
to the embryonic age at which the microsurgical manipulation
occurs (see Figs. 1-15 and 1-16).

     In another series of experiments investigating epithelio-
mesenchymal tissue interactions, trypsin, which is a proteo-
lytic enzyme, was used to study the effects of disruption of
these tissue interactions at different time points in
embryonic development of explanted inner ears. Trypsin has
been shown to disrupt normal "in vitro" morphogenesis of
several organ anlagen which normally exhibit branching morphogenesis. In our experimental series, trypsin treatment
of otic explants interfered with the expression of the normal
pattern of inner ear development "in vitro". There was a
direct correlation between the embryonic age at time of
exposure to trypsin and the severity of dismorphogenesis of
the inner ear. The earlier explants were most profoundly
affected, with both vestibular and auditory portions of the
inner ear being abnormal; whereas, with increasing embryonic
age, abnormalities of inner ear development were confined to
the auditory portions of the inner ear. The results suggest
that integrity of the otocyst basal lamina and intercommuni-
cation between mesenchyme cells are important factors in early
otic development. The major effect of trypsin on inner ear
morphogenesis is thought to be through disruption of epithelio-
mesenchymal tissue interactions which may act to regulate the
progressive expression of early otic development (Fig. 1-17).

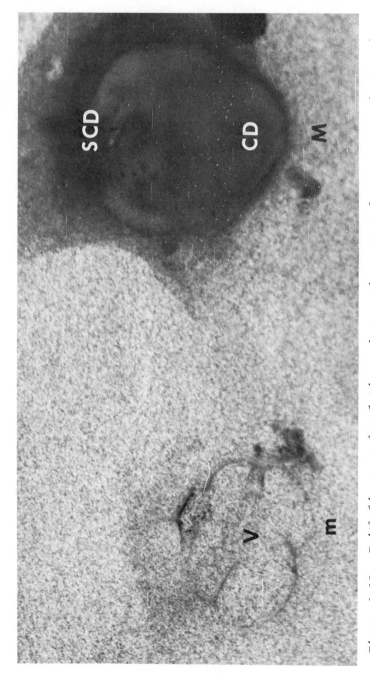

Figure 1-15. Epithelio-mesenchymal tissue interaction. 10.5 day otocyst explants, nine days in vitro. Left otocyst (reduced mesenchyme) exhibits total dysmorphogenesis; right otocyst (normal mesenchyme) normal otic morphogenesis. (X180)

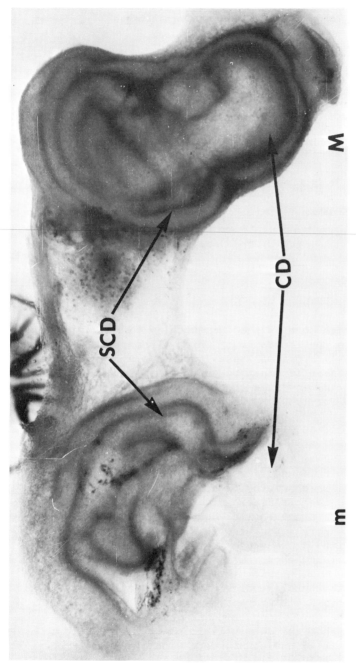

Figure 1-16. Epithelio-mesenchymal tissue interaction. 12 day otocyst explants, eight days in vitro. Left otocyst (reduced mesenchyme) normal development of semicircular ducts and utricle with dysmorphogenesis limited to the area of the saccule and cochlea. Right otocyst (normal mesenchyme – normal otic morphogenesis. (XI80)

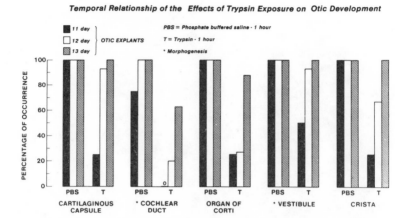

Figure 1-17. A histogram depicting the effects of trypsin exposure on in vitro otic development.

GENETIC MUTANTS

There are more than 50 genetically different strains of deaf mice (Deol, 1980), of which a number has been studied histologically. One of these, the Kreisler strain of mice, is of particular interest in that the malformation of homozygotes (kr/kr) involves the entire bony and membranous labyrinth (Hertwig, 1944). The cell kinetics of the otocyst epithelium of the homozygotic Kreisler embryos has been documented (Ruben, 1973) and found to be abnormal with respect to otocysts of heterozygotic littermates and a normal strain of mice (CBA-J). The expression of the labyrinthine lesion in the Kreisler mouse is variable. Some ears will have only a large cyst which can be of sufficient size as to compromise and compress the brainstem (Fig. 1-18), while other inner ears will have a near normal bony labyrinth but will be devoid of sensory structures. This variability of genetic expression into a phenotype must be taken into account in studies involving the Kreisler mouse inner ear.

Ultrastructural studies of brain/otocyst relationships of homozygotic Kreisler embryos (kr/kr) show a greater separation of the developing otic anlage and the adjacent rhombencephalon than that which is found in the normal mouse (Fig. 1-19). This finding is congruent with previous light microscopic studies (Deol, 1964, 1966, 1980). These observations

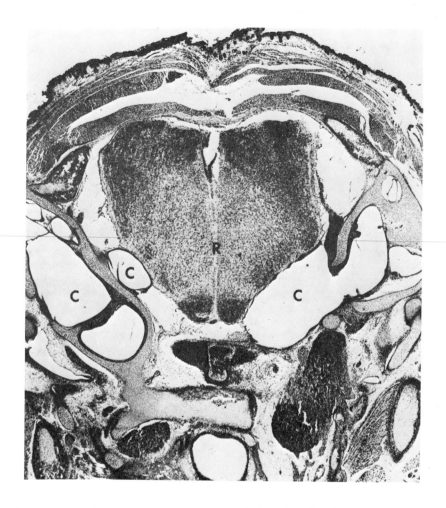

Fig. 1-18. A cross section through the head of a newborn homozygotic Kreisler (kr/kr) mouse showing the severity of the dysmorphogenesis of the inner ear in this mutant. Cysts of inner ear origin are seen compressing the rhombencephalon.

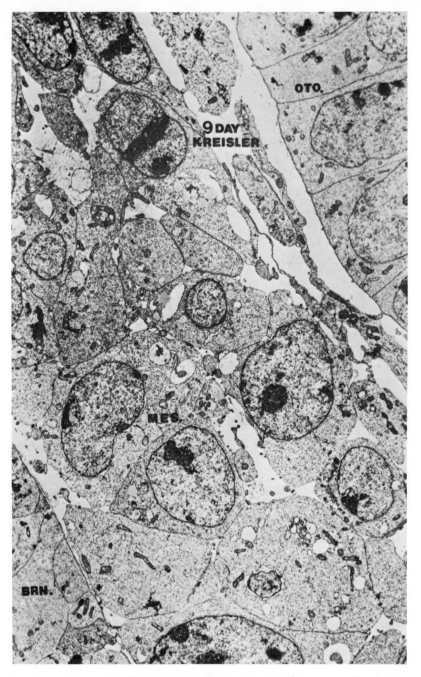

Figure 1-19. An electron micrograph of the area of closest apposition between the otocyst and rhombencephalon of a 23 somite homozygotic Kreisler embryo. The separation between these two neuroepithelial tissues is over 100 times the normal distance.

would suggest that the site of gene action may not only be within the inner ear anlagen, but a combination of factors.

To further examine this hypothesis, a series of studies was undertaken to study the effect of interacting normal (CBA-J) brain with homozygotic Kreisler (kr/kr) otocysts and, conversely, homozygotic Kreisler (kr/kr) brain with normal (CBA-J) otocysts. These experiments were performed "in vitro" by explanting an otocyst of either a normal or mutant geno-type and allowing it to develop in direct contact with a rhombencephalon explant of either a normal or mutant geno-type. The experiments are difficult to perform because of the low fertility of the Kreisler strain of mice and, con-sequently, these experiments must be carried out over a number of years. Additionally, any interpretation of the results must take into account the variability of the phenotypic expression of the Kreisler inner ear malformation. This requires that a large number of studies be done which further extends the length of time which is needed for this particular series of experiments. Preliminary findings show that a homo-zygotic Kreisler (kr/kr) otocyst will develop less abnormally when interacted with a normal (CBA-J) rhombencephalon. Addi-tionally, there appears to be little or no effect on the "in vitro" pattern of normal (CBA-J) otocyst development when interacted with homozygotic Kreisler (kr/kr) rhombencephalon in comparison to normal otocysts interacted with normal rhombencephalon.

The ultrastructural and organ culture studies indicate that the mode of gene action on development of the inner ear of the Kreisler (kr/kr) mouse may be indirect. Gene action may be on a combination of tissues (only the brain has been studied), which in turn, interact to cause abnormality in the pattern of gene expression of the developing otocyst. These findings on embryogenesis of the Kreisler (kr/kr) inner ear are congruent with our embryologic findings on the factors which control the normal expression of gene action in the developmental program of the inner ear, e.g., interactions among rhombencephalon, mesenchyme, and the otic anlage.

These preliminary observations are useful in furthering our understanding of genetic disease of the inner ear, as they suggest that some genetic abnormalities may not directly affect the inner ear, but may be the result of abnormalities interfering with the expression of the normal sequence of inductive tissue interactions which direct the formation of the inner ear. This type of mechanism may be operant in a genetic syndrome which is associated with other abnormalities; e.g., Waardenburg's Disease, Apert's Disease, Pendred's Disease, etc. This, then, allows the investigator to focus attention on what could be a common mechanism which could result in a heterogenous phenotype instead of focusing on the description of abnormalities of the inner ear.

CONCLUSION

The study of the development of the inner ear has made many advances over the past few years. Knowledge is now available concerning some of the mechanisms of the normal sequential genetic control of differentiation of the ear. This information has given substance to the hypothesis of two possible mechanisms for genetic disease of the inner ear; either a direct or a secondary effect which could be due to abnormalities in inductive tissue interactions that control the expression of the development of the inner ear (Fig. 1-20). These observations should enable a more direct investigation of the biochemical abnormalities which underly genetic sensory-neural deafness in man which would express themselves both pre and postpartum. Understanding of these diseases would allow the otologist to possibly institute interventions which would result in the prevention of deafness.

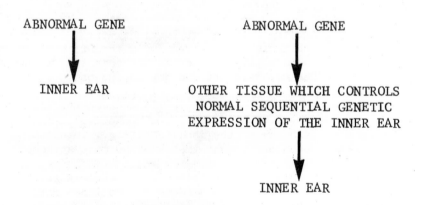

Figure 1-20. Two possible modes of gene action in the production of a malformed labyrinth.

ACKNOWLEDGEMENTS

The authors express their gratitude for assistance in the preparation of this manuscript to: Susan Montalvo (typing and proofreading), Linval Montfries (illustrations), and Akira Suzuka (electron microscopy).

REFERENCES

Deol, M.S. "The abnormalities of the inner ear in Kreisler mice" Journal of Embryology and Experimental Morphology 12:475-490, 1964.

Deol, M.S. "Influence of the neural tube on the differentiation of the inner ear in the mammalian embryo" Nature 209:219-220, 1966.

Deol, M.S. "Genetic malformations of the inner ear in mouse and man" in Gorlin, R.J. (ed.) Morphogenesis and Malformation of the Ear. Birth Defects: Original Article Series, Vol. XVI No. 4, (New York: Allan R. Liss, Inc.), 1980.

Fraser, G.R. The Causes of Profound Deafness in Childhood (London: Bailliere-Tindal), 1976.

Held, H. Untersuchungen über den feineren Bau des Ohrlabyrinthes der Wirbelthiere: II Zur Entwicklungsgeschichte des Cortischen Organs und der Macula Acustica bei Sangethieren und Vogeln. Abhandl. d. math. phys. K.d.k. sachs. Gesellsch.d.Wissensch. (Leipzig) 31:193-293, 1909.

Hertwig, P. "Die geneses der hirn und gehörganmissifildungen fei röntgenmutierten Kreisler-mausen" Z. Mensch. Vereb. Konst. 28:327-354, 1944.

Li, C.W., Van De Water, T.R. and Ruben, R.J. "The fate mapping of the eleventh and twelfth day mouse otocyst: an 'in vitro' study of the sites of origin of the embryonic inner ear sensory structures" Journal of Morphology 157:249-268, 1978.

Retzius, M.G. Das Gehörorgan der Wirbelthiere (Stockholm: Samson and Wallin), 1881-1884.

Ruben, R.J. "Development of the inner ear of the mouse: A
    radioautographic study of terminal mitoses" Acta
    Otolaryngologica Supplement 220:1-44, 1967.

Ruben, R.J. "Development and cell kinetics for the Kreisler
    (kr/kr) mouse" Laryngoscope 83:1440-1468, 1973.

Ruben, R.J. and Kruger, B. "Hearing loss in the elderly"
    in Katzman, R. and Terry R. (eds.) Neurology of Aging.
    Contemporary Neurl. Series (F.A. Davis & Co.) In
    preparation.

Sher, A.E. "The embryonic and postnatal development of the
    inner ear of the mouse" Acta Otolaryngologica Supplement
    285:1-77, 1971.

Van De Water, T.R. "Effects of the statoacoustic ganglion
    complex upon the growing otocyst" Annals of Otology,
    Rhinology and Laryngology, Supplement (33)85:1-32,
    1976.

Van De Water, T.R., Heywood, P. and Ruben, R.J. "Development
    of sensory structures in organ cultures of the twelfth
    and thirteenth gestation day mouse embryo inner ears"
    Annals of Otology, Rhinology and Laryngology, Supplement
    4, 82:1-19, 1973.

Van De Water, T.R. and Ruben, R.J. "Organ culture of the
    mammalian inner ear" Acta Otolaryngologica 71:303-312,
    1971.

Van De Water, T.R. and Ruben, R.J. "Quantification of the
    'in vitro' development of the mouse embryo inner ear"
    Annals of Otology, Rhinology and Laryngology, Supple-
    ment 4, 82:19-21, 1973.

FIGURE LEGEND

A   - Ampulla

BM   - Basement Membrane

BRN.   - Brain Stem

C   - Cystic Inner Ear

CD   - Cochlear Duct

CV   - Coated Vesicle

ECM   - Extracellular Matrix

MES., M - Normal Mesenchyme Explant, Mesenchyme Cells

m   - Reduced Mesenchyme Explant

N   - Notochord

OTO., O - Otocyst

OC   - Otic Cup

OP   - Otic Placode

R   - Rhombencephalon

SCD   - Semicircular Duct

V   - Vesicular Form

VIIn   - Facio-Statoacoustic Ganglion

(+)   - With Ganglion Explant

(-)   - Without Ganglion Explant

ANATOMY OF THE INNER EAR

I. Hunter-Duvar
University of Toronto, Toronto, Ontario

The mammalian inner ear has the dual function of being
the sensory end organ for hearing and for equilibrium. Whereas
electrophysiological tests for newborn and older infants can
isolate electrical responses from the hearing system, responses to behavioral tests of hearing may require functioning
of both systems.

There are substantial data to indicate that the human
cochlea is anatomically developed and able to respond to
auditory stimuli by the seventh month of gestation (Bast and
Anson, 1949; Bredberg, 1966; Fleischer, 1955; Lorente de No,
1926; Wedenberg, 1965). In humans electrophysiological
responses to auditory stimuli are thus available at birth
(full term). Behavioral responses to auditory stimuli are
available providing the response solicited comes from a
system that is also functioning at birth. It follows that,
the simpler the response required, the less is the danger
of misinterpreting pathology in another system as cochlear
pathology.

It is to be expected that although the human auditory
system is available at birth it is largely functionally
undifferentiated, and changes in threshold and added ability
to discriminate auditory stimuli will occur with differentiation. There is evidence that with auditory deprivation or
nonuse the system does not completely differentiate with
resulting pathology (Babighian et al., 1973; Trune, 1978,
1981). Many of the data relative to development of auditory
capability have come from animal experimentation. It should
not be surprising to find differences in electrophysiological
and behavioral capabilities of the auditory system of newborn
humans and certain newborn animals (e.g., cat) since the
former is anatomically developed at birth and the latter is
not.

Like the cochlea the vestibular portion of the human
inner ear is anatomically developed at birth. Vestibular

reflexes are present and the newborn is capable of orienting responses. This capability makes possible reliable behavioral tests of hearing in infants.

This chapter is devoted to a description of the normal anatomy of the inner ear. It is hoped the understanding of the function of the inner ear and of pathological changes to its function may be aided by a knowledge of the structure.

MEMBRANOUS LABYRINTH

The membranous labyrinth lies in the bony labyrinth of the temporal bone and contains the sensory epithelia of both the vestibular and cochlear systems (Fig. 2-1). The membranous labyrinth contains endolymphatic fluid and is largely surrounded by perilymphatic fluid. Sensory epithelia of the vestibule and the ampullae of the semicircular canals are innervated by the vestibular branch of the VIIIth nerve and the cochlea is innervated by the cochlear portion of the VIIIth nerve.

Vestibular Sensory Epithelium

The sensory epithelia of the mammalian vestibular system consist of the macula saccule, macula utricle, and the cristae in the ampullae of anterior, posterior, and lateral semi-circular canals. The saccule and utricle are otolith organs and are largely responsible for the detection of linear acceleration. The cristae have their sensors covered by the cupulae and are generally responsible for the detection of angular acceleration. The vestibular sensory detectors consist of two types of specialized cells known as type I and type II hair cells. These differ in both shape and innervation (Fig. 2-2). The type I cell is generally flask-shaped and surrounded by a calyx which is the ending of an afferent nerve fiber (Figs. 2-2, 2-3). Type II hair cells are generally rod-shaped and innervated by small afferent and efferent nerve endings (Figs. 2-2, 2-4). Both type I and type II cells contain 20 to 100 stereocilia(s) of staggered length and one longer kinocilium(k) on their surfaces (Fig. 2-5). They are usually surrounded by supporting cells and have a circular nucleus located in the lower half of the cell (Fig. 2-2).

In the macula utricle the hair cells are oriented with their kinocilia facing inward toward a less dense strip of cells with shorter stereocilia known as the striola (Fig. 2-6).

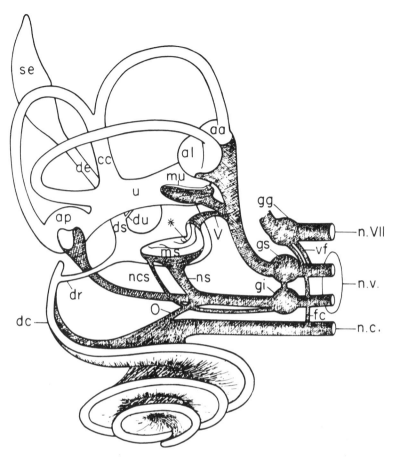

Figure 2-1. Diagram showing the membranous labyrinth and the general plan of innervation of the sensory regions in the inner ear in mammals. ms - macula saccule; V - Voits' nerve; ncs - cochlea saccular nerve; ns - saccular nerve; mu - macula utricle; aa - anterior ampulla; ap - posterior ampulla; al - lateral ampulla; cc - crus commune; ds - saccular duct; du - utricular duct; se - endolymphatic sac; de - endolymphatic duct; dr - ductus reuniens; dc - cochlear duct; nVII - facial nerve; nv - vestibular nerve; nc - cochlear nerve; gs - superior vestibular ganglion; gi - inferior vestibular ganglion; gg - geniculate ganglion; 0 - anastomosis of Oort; fc - facio-cochlear anastomosis; vf - vestibulo-facial anastomosis (adapted from H.H. Lindeman; Morphology of Vestibular Sensory Regions, Advances in Anatomy, Embryology and Cell Biology. New York, Springer Verlag, 42: 1, 1969, with permission.)

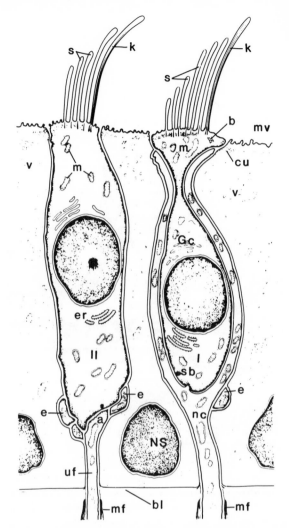

Figure 2-2. *Schematic drawing illustrating the general structure of the vestibular sensory epithelium. Type I cell (I) is flask-shaped and is almost completely surrounded by a nerve chalice (nc). Type II cell (II) is rod-shaped and is innervated by small afferent (a) and efferent (e) nerve endings. Many stereocilia (s) and one kinocilium (k) protrude from the free surface of each sensory cell. Microvilli (mv) are found on the surface of sensory and supporting cells. b - basal body; cu - cuticular plate; m - mitochondria; Gc - Golgi complex; er - endoplasmic reticulum; sb - synaptic bar; v - cytoplasmic vesicles; uf - unmyelinated fiber; mf - myelinated fiber; NS - nucleus of supporting cell; bl - basal lamina.*

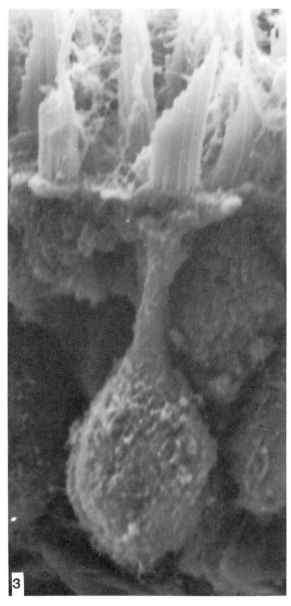

Figure 2-3. Scanning micrograph showing flask-shaped type I cell of macula saccule.

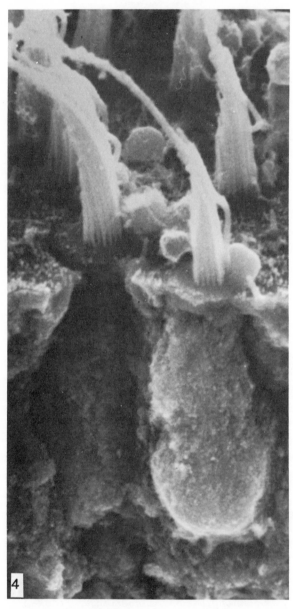

Figure 2-4. Scanning micrograph of rod-shaped type II cell of macula saccule.

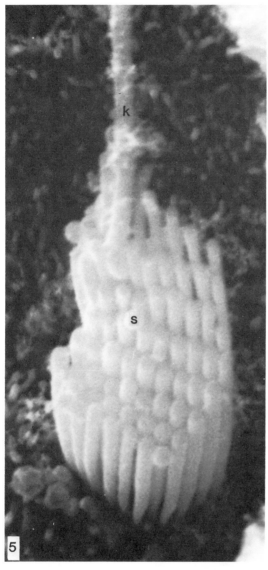

Figure 2-5. Scanning micrograph of surface of a vestibular sensory cell demonstrating the staggered formation of the stereocilia (s) and the longer kinocilium (k). Debris on the kinocilium indicate attachment to the intermediate mesh.

43

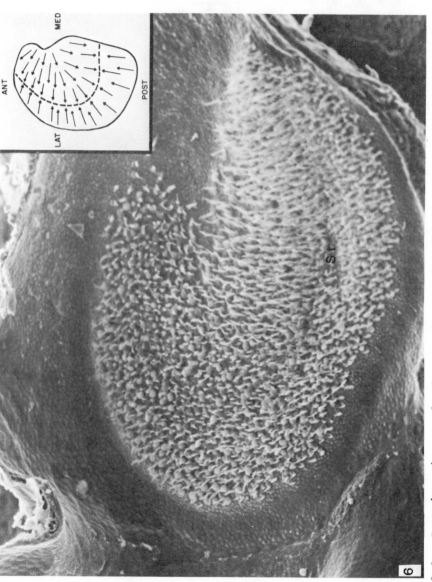

Figure 2-6. Scanning micrograph of a macula utricle with the statoconial membrane removed demonstrating the typical shell-shape formed by the sensory cells. The striola (St) are seen to take the general pattern shown in the inset which shows the polarization or orientation of the sensory cells. In the macula utricle, kinocilium direction is toward the striola.

44

A similar area is also seen in the macula saccule; however, the hair cells are oriented with their kinocilia and longest stereocilia facing away from the striola (Fig. 2-7). The stereocilia on the hair cells of the otolith organs are surrounded by an intermediate mesh which is attached to the kinocilia and which carries a layer of otoconia on its upper surface (Fig. 2-8). It is the inertia of these statoconia, relative to the macula, which is the stimulus for the detection of linear acceleration (Wilson and Melvill Jones, 1979).

A saddle-shaped crista (Fig. 2-9) is located in each ampulla at the end of anterior, posterior, and lateral semicircular canals (Fig. 2-1). The hair cells on the surface of each crista are all polarized in the same direction. In the lateral crista kinocilia and longest stereocilia face toward the utricle, whereas in the anterior and posterior crista they face away from the utricle. There is considerable difference in length of stereocilia on hair cells and density of hair cells over the surface of the crista. The central area is less densely populated and contains cells with shorter, thicker stereocilia (Fig. 2-9). The cilia of each crista are covered with a fibrous gelatinous mass called the cupula (Fig. 2-10). The cupula which ordinarily extends to the outer borders of the ampulla is subject to severe shrinkage during histological preparation due to removal of its fluid content. Movement of the cupula by the endolymph of the vestibular canals is considered to be the stimulus for detection of angular acceleration.

THE MEMBRANOUS COCHLEA

The membranous cochlea is continuous with the vestibule and is joined to it at the ductus reuniens (Fig. 2-1). This junction lies in the area beneath the footplate of the stapes which occupies the oval window (Fig. 2-11). The human membranous cochlea spirals like a corkscrew for two and one half turns and it is surrounded by bone on all sides (Figs. 2-11, 2-12). The central bony shaft collects the fibers of the cochlear nerve as they converge from the sensory cells distributed along the organ of Corti which extends from the base to the apex of the cochlea (Fig. 2-12). The outer bony wall encompasses the perilymphatic fluid spaces of scala vestibuli and scala tympani as well as the spiral ligament of scala media (Figs. 2-11, 2-12).

Reissner's membrane separates the perilymph of the scala vestibuli from the endolymph of the scala media. This

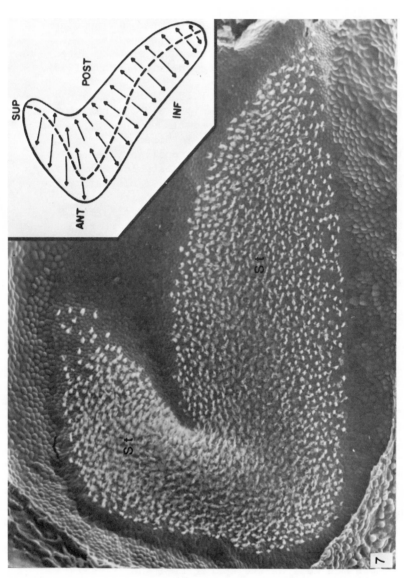

Figure 2-7. Scanning micrograph of the hook-shaped macula saccule with the statoconial membrane removed. The striola (St) can be seen as shown in the inset which depicts the orientation of the sensory cells. In the saccule, the kinocilium and longest stereocilia face away from the striola.

46

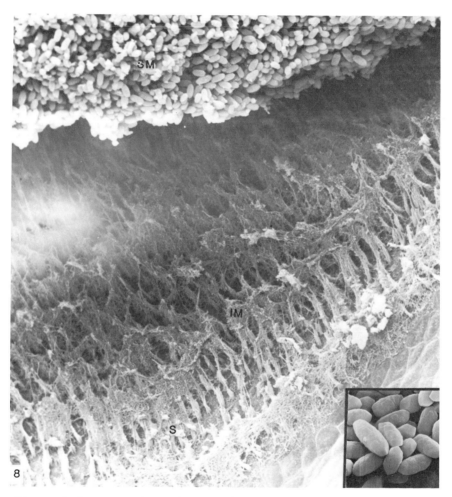

Figure 2-8. Scanning micrograph of an area where the stato-conial membrane (SM) has been elevated to show the inter-mediate mesh (IM) which attaches it to the sensory cells (S) of macula utricle and macula saccule. The inset is a higher power micrograph showing individual otoliths of the stato-conial membrane.

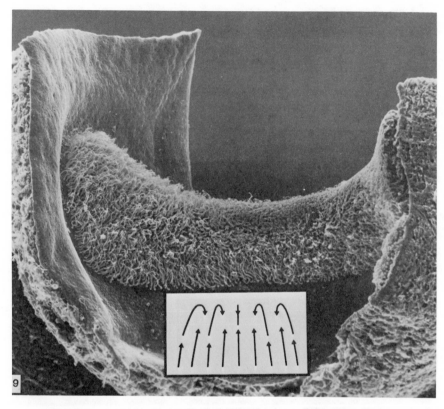

Figure 2-9. A scanning micrograph showing the sensory epithelium of the saddle-shaped crista. Cilia are shorter and thicker on the sensory cells covering the central area of the crista. The population of sensory cells is also less dense in this area. Polarization of the sensory cells is depicted in the inset. In the crista the kinocilia are all oriented in the same direction.

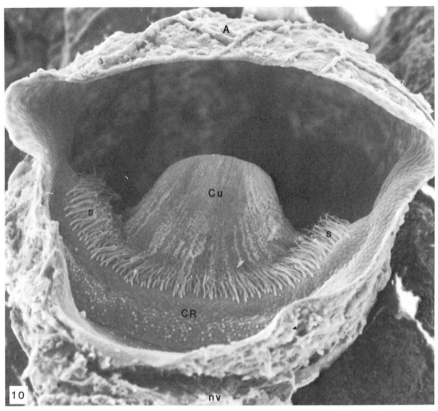

Figure 2-10. A scanning micrograph of an ampulla (A) partly cut away to show the crista (CR) and the cupula (Cu). The gelatinous cupula, which is considered to cover all the sensory cells (S) and extend to the walls of the ampulla, is shrunken to a fraction of its reputed size because the specimens must be completely dried for SEM inspection. A portion of the vestibular nerve (nv) can be seen at the bottom of the micrograph where it enters the ampulla.

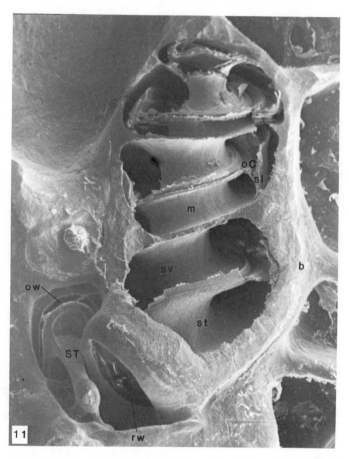

Figure 2-11. Bone (b) has been removed from the cochlea and
the scanning micrograph shows the relationship of the vestibule which lies beneath the stapes (ST) and the oval window
(ow). The vestibule leads directly into the scala vestibuli
(sv). The bony modiolus (m) containing the auditory nerve
is seen to occupy the center portion of the cochlea with the
membranous cochlea containing the organ of Corti (oC) and
the spiral ligament (sl) spiraling around it. rw - round
window; st - scala tympani.

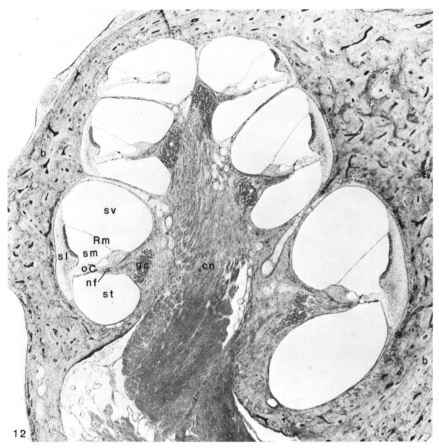

Figure 2-12. A light micrograph of a thick section through the cochlea shows how nerve fibers (nf) from the membranous cochlea run to the cochlear nerve (cn) located in the modiolus. Reissner's membrane (Rm) separating scala vestibuli (sv) from scala media (sm) is clearly seen. Bone (b) is seen to surround the scala and the spiral ligament (sl). oC - organ of Corti; gc - ganglion cells; st - scala tympani.

membrane is a two cell layer with mesodermal cells adjacent
to perilymph (Fig. 2-13) and ectodermal cells in contact with
the endolymph (Fig. 2-14).

Cochlear Sensory Epithelium

The sensory epithelium of the membranous cochlea is contained within the scala media. The tectorial membrane -
a gelatinous, fibrous mass - overlies the sensory hair cells
which are contained in the organ of Corti. The upper side of
the tectorial membrane has a distinct fibrous pattern when
seen in its dehydrated state (Fig. 2-15). Evidence of firm
contact between the tallest stereocilia of the outer hair
cells and the underside of the tectorial membrane is clearly
displayed in the "W" imprints in Hardesty's membrane (Fig.
2-16). No such definitive contact is seen for stereocilia
of inner hair cells.

The sensory receptors for hearing - or "hair cells" -
are contained in the organ of Corti. This epithelial ridge
rests on the basilar membrane and extends from the base to
the apex of the cochlear duct (Figs. 2-11, 2-17).

Cochlear hair cells are of two distinct types. There
are generally three (sometimes four) rows of outer hair cells
and a single row of inner hair cells (Fig. 2-18). Inner and
outer hair cell populations are separated by supporting
cells, known as pillar cells, and by the tunnel of Corti, a
relatively large fluid space formed by inner and outer pillar
cells (Figs. 2-17, 2-19).

Outer hair cells are long cylindrical cells with a circular nucleus located in the basal area of the cell (Figs.
2-17, 2-19). The top of the outer hair cell is largely covered by a dense cuticular plate which supports approximately
one hundred long specialized microvilli called stereocilia.
This tuft of hair-like structures typically assumes a W shape
on the top of the outer hair cell (Fig. 2-20). Outer hair
cells are surrounded by fluid and are supported at base and
apex by Deiters cells (Figs. 2-17, 2-19). They are innervated at the basal end by a large number of afferent and
efferent nerve endings (Fig. 2-21). These are the enlarged
ends of fibers which travel across the tunnel of Corti and
through the habenula perforata to the modiolus (Figs. 2-17,
2-22, 2-23).

The inner hair cells are located in a single row on the
modiolar side of the pillar cells (Fig. 2-18). They have a

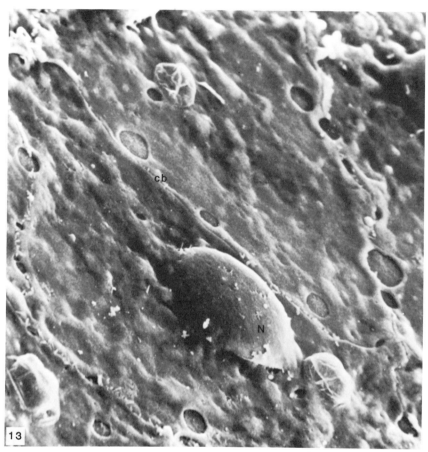

Figure 2-13. A scanning micrograph shows the mesothelial cell layer on the upper surface of Reissner's membrane. These thin cells have large nuclei (N) which appear as bumps on the surface of each cell. cb - cell border.

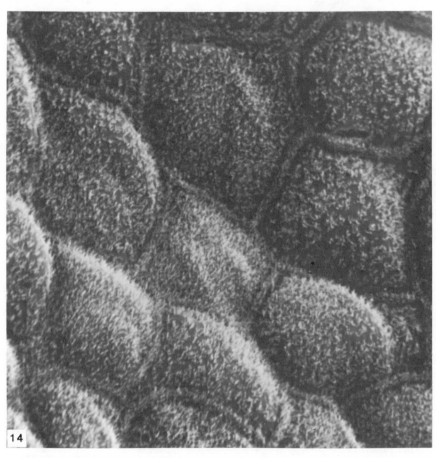

Figure 2-14. A scanning micrograph of the underside of Reissner's membrane showing the endothelial cells which face the endolymph of the scala media. Cells have well defined borders and large populations of microvilli.

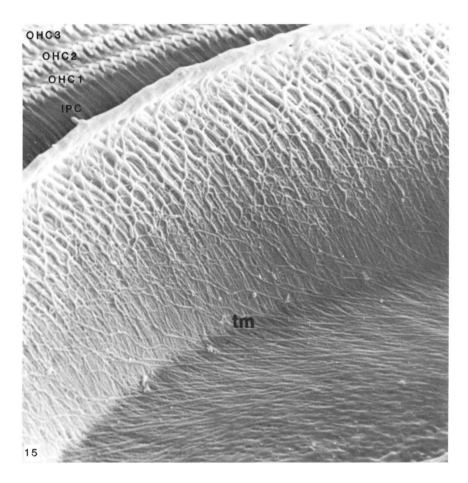

Figure 2-15. A scanning micrograph of the upper side of the tectorial membrane (tm) after critical point drying demonstrates the fibrous nature of the membrane. IPC - headplates of inner pillar cells; OHCL - stereocilia of the first row of outer hair cells.

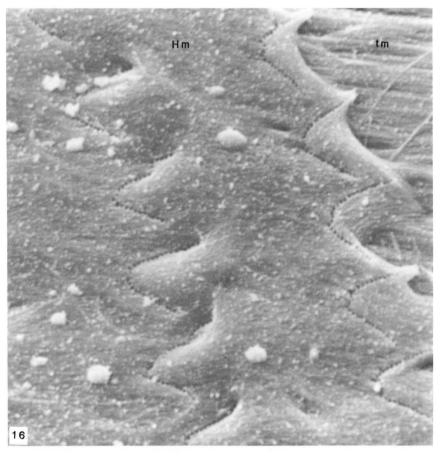

Figure 2-16. A scanning micrograph of a portion of the underside of the tectorial membrane (tm) shows imprints in Hardesty's membrane (Hm) from the tallest stereocilia of the outer hair cells.

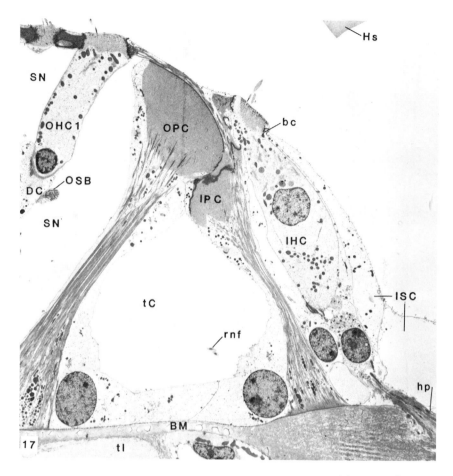

Figure 2-17. A transmission micrograph of a thin section through part of the organ of Corti demonstrating the typical location of first row outer hair cells (OHC1) and inner hair cells (IHC). They are separated by the outer pillar cells (OPC) and inner pillar cells (IPC) which together form the fluid space known as the tunnel of Corti (tC). Outer hair cells are supported by Deiters cells (DC) and surrounded by the fluid in spaces of Nuel (SN); whereas, inner hair cells are surrounded by the inner pillar cells and border cells (bc). Hs - stripe of Hensen on tectorial membrane; OSB - first outer spiral bundle of nerve fibers; rnf - radial nerve fibers; ISC - inner sulcus cells; hp - habenula perforata; BM - basilar membrane; tl - tympanic layer cells.

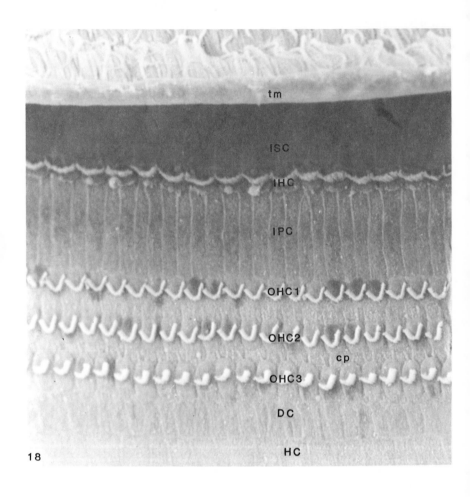

tm

ISC

IHC

IPC

OHC1

OHC2

cp

OHC3

DC

HC

18

Figure 2-18. Scanning micrograph of the organ of Corti shows the surface areas of the various cells. tm - tectorial membrane; ISC - inner sulcus cells; IHC - stereocilia and tops of inner hair cells; IPC - headplates of inner pillar cells; OHC (1, 2, 3) - W shapes of stereocilia on three rows of outer hair cells; cp - cuticular surface of the phalangeal processes of Deiters cells; DC - Deiters cells; HC - Hensen cells.

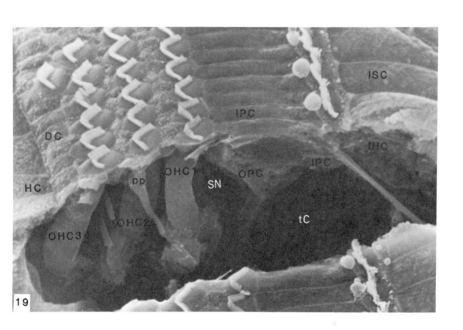

Figure 2-19. Scanning micrograph of a shrinkage crack in the organ of Corti shows both the upper surface and interior structural aspects. HC - Hensen cells; DC - Deiters cells; OHC (1, 2, 3) - stereocilia and cell bodies of three rows of outer hair cells; pp - phalangeal process of Deiters cell; SN - space of Nuel; IPC - inner pillar cell; OPC - outer pillar cell; tC - tunnel of Corti; IHC - inner hair cell; ISC - inner sulcus cell.

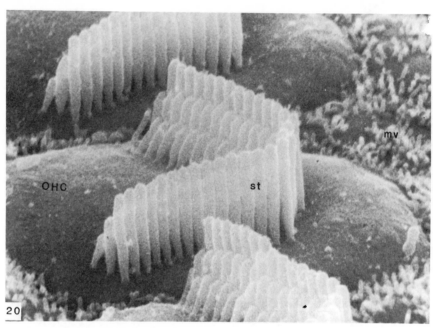

Figure 2-20. A scanning micrograph showing the arrangement of stereocilia (st) on outer hair cells (OHC). mv - microvilli.

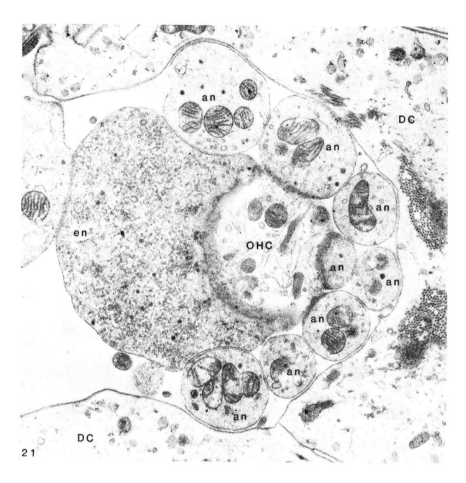

Figure 2-21. A transmission micrograph of a thin section cut horizontally through the basal tip of an outer hair cell (OHC) demonstrating the arrangement of nerve endings. Both efferent (en) and afferent nerve endings (an) are seen in contact with the hair cell as well as in contact with each other. DC - Deiters cell.

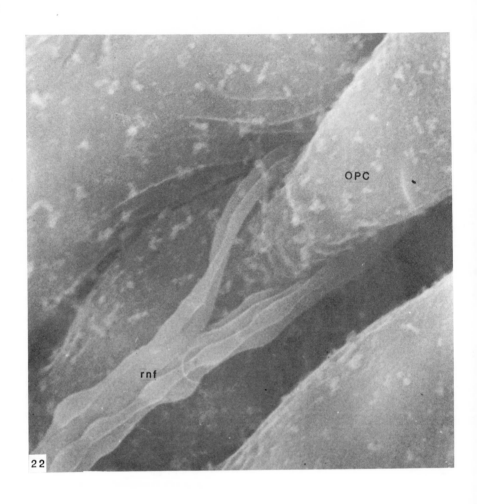

Figure 2-22. A scanning micrograph showing radial nerve fibers (rnf) crossing the tunnel of Corti and going around an outer pillar cell (OPC) as they travel between the tunnel spiral bundle and the outer spiral bundles.

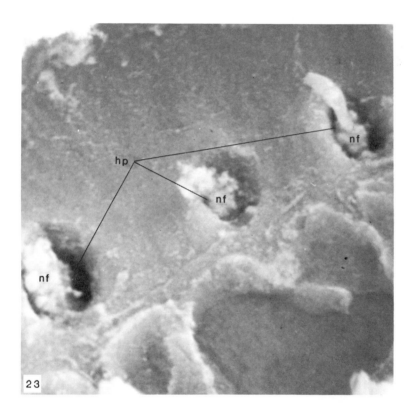

Figure 2-23. A scanning micrograph shows nerve fibers (nf) broken off as they travel through the habenula perforata (hp).

centrally located nucleus and are completely surrounded by
supporting cells (Fig. 2-17). Stereocilia of inner hair
cells generally consist of one row of tall cilia in a curve
with two or more rows of quite short cilia behind (Fig. 2-24).
Inner hair cells are innervated at the base by afferent nerve
endings, and the inner hair cell population receives approximately ninety-five percent of the afferent innervation of the
cochlea.

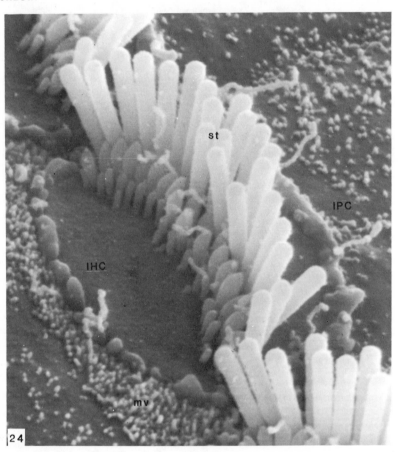

*Figure 2-24. Scanning micrograph demonstrating the arrange-
ment of stereocilia (st) on the surface of an inner hair
cell (IHC). IPC - inner pillar cell; mv - microvilli.*

The architecture of the organ of Corti is delicately
complex (Fig. 2-25). Hensen cells cover the lateral aspect
of the organ and join to Deiters cells upon which rest the

basal ends of the hair cells (Figs. 2-17, 2-25). The long
phalangeal processes of the Deiters cells extend to the surface of the organ of Corti and form the reticular lamina
which supports and separates the apical ends of the second
and third row of outer hair cells (Figs. 2-19, 2-26). The
hair cell bodies are separated from each other, from the
phalangeal processes of the Deiters cells, and from the
outer pillar cells by the fluid filled spaces of Nuel (Figs.
2-19, 2-25). Fibril filled portions of the inner pillar
cells extend over the heads of the outer pillar cells and
become the surface area of the pillar cells in the sub-
tectorial space (Fig. 2-17). They also extend between the
tops of the first row of outer hair cells and form that portion of the reticular lamina. The inner hair cells are surrounded and supported by the inner pillar cells and the border
cells of the inner spiral sulcus (Fig. 2-17). The organ of
Corti is bounded on the modiolar side by the inner sulcus
cells and the spiral limbus, and on the other side by
Claudius cells and the cells of the spiral prominence (Fig.
2-25). The whole structure rests on the basilar membrane
(Fig. 2-25).

The basilar membrane separates the endolymphatic scala
media from the perilymphatic scala tympani. It is widest at
the apical (low frequency) end of the cochlea and narrowest
at the basal (high frequency) end. It is composed largely
of fiber bundles which are densely packed at the basal end
and loosely packed at the apical end (Fig. 27a, b). The
underside of the basilar membrane is covered by a layer of
mesothelial cells which are in contact with the perilymph
of the scala tympani (Fig. 2-28).

                        OTOTOXIC INSULT

The cochlea is subject to damage from many sources among
which are acoustic trauma, ototoxic drugs, viral infection,
and congenital malfunction. Much research must be done
before definitive statements can be made about anatomical
correlates of cochlear insult. Experimental results are
clouded by tremendous inter-subject variability as well as
species variability in susceptibility to insult.

Generally, sensory cells are more susceptible than
supporting cells to damage (Figs. 2-29, 2-31). Once the
sensory cells are lost or damaged they are never replaced.
Fortunately a large measure of functional overlap appears to

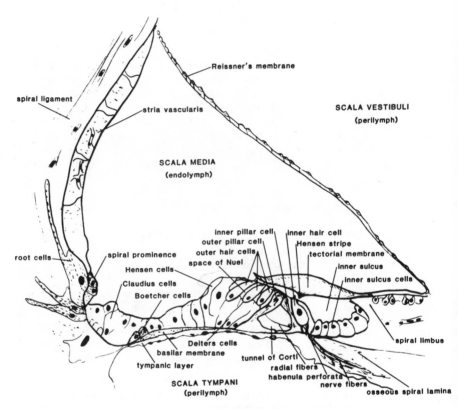

Figure 2-25. A schematic drawing of a cross section through the membranous cochlea showing the architecture and the relationship of various cells and fluid spaces.

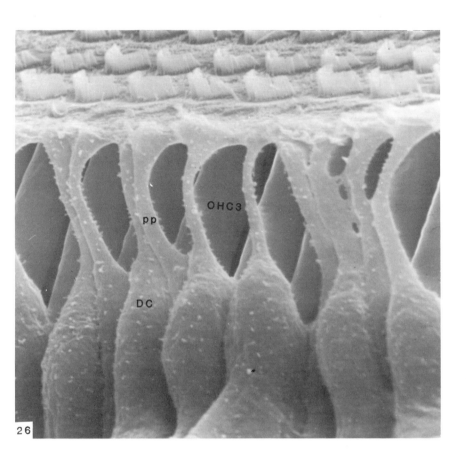

Figure 2-26. A scanning micrograph showing the relationship of Deiters cells (DC) and thier phalangeal processes (pp) to the third row of outer hair cells (OHC3). The organ of Corti has been separated along the Hensen - Deiters cell border.

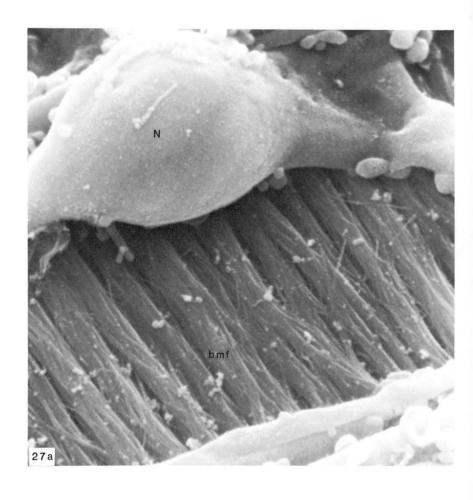

Figure 2-27a. A scanning micrograph shows the fibers of the basilar membrane (bmf) in the lower middle turn of the cochlea. N - nucleus of tympanic layer cell.

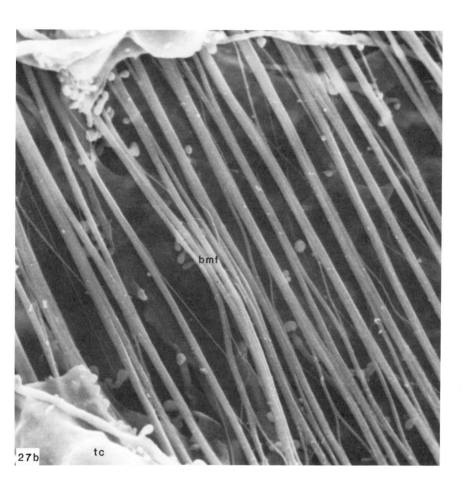

Figure 2-27b. Compares the basilar membrane fibers in the apical turn of the cochlea. tc - edge of tympanic layer cell.

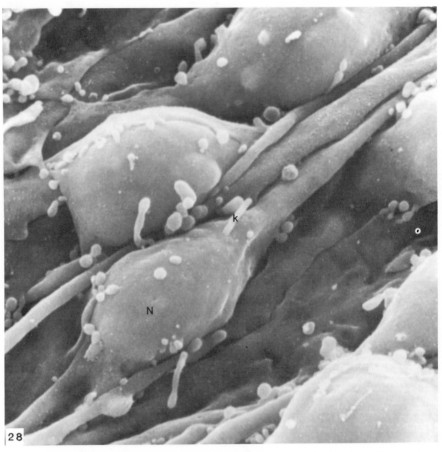

Figure 2-28. A scanning micrograph of mesothelial cells of the tympanic layer which cover the underside of the basilar membrane and contact the perilymph of the scala tympani. N - nucleus; k - kinocilium.

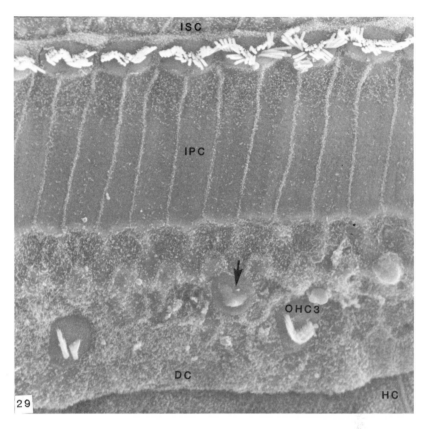

Figure 2-29. A scanning micrograph of the surface of the organ of Corti several days after acoustic overstimulation. Outer hair cells are almost completely destroyed in this area with only two damaged third row cells (OHC3) remaining. One severely damaged outer hair cell with completely fused stereocilia can be seen in the second row (arrow). Deiters cells (DC) have overgrown and largely maintained the shape of the organ of Corti. Inner hair cells are seen to remain although the stereocilia on most are in great disarray. The headplates of the inner pillar cells (IPC) are undamaged as are the inner sulcus cells (ISC) and Hensen cells (HC).

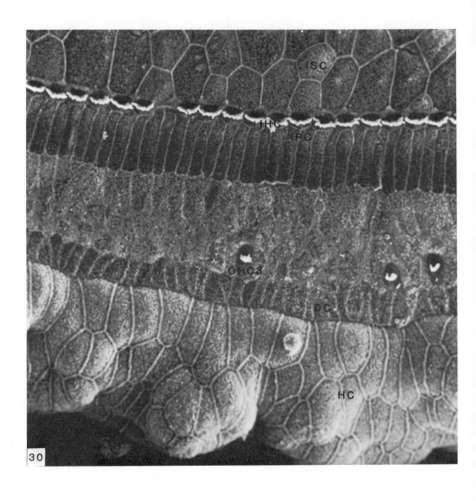

Figure 2-30. Scanning micrograph of the organ of Corti from the middle turn of a cochlea subjected to damage from an ototoxic antibiotic. Outer hair cells are almost completely eliminated with only three damaged cells of the third row (OHC3) remaining. Inner hair cells (IHC) and their stereocilia appear almost intact in the area. Supporting cells have maintained the structure although Hensen cells (HC) are considerably distorted. Some damage can be seen to the ends of the headplates of the inner pillar cells (IPC). ISC - inner sulcus cells; DC - Deiters cells.

72

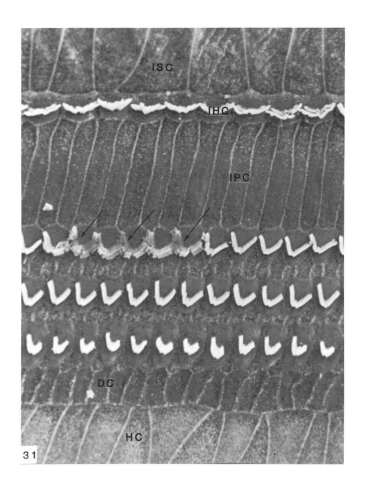

Figure 2-31. Scanning micrograph of surface area of the organ
of Corti a few hours after acoustic overstimulation showing
disarray of stereocilia on the first row of outer hair cells
(arrows). All other structures have their normal appearance.
ISC - inner sulcus cells; IPC - inner pillar cells; DC -
Deiters cells; HC - Hensen cells; IHC - inner hair cells.

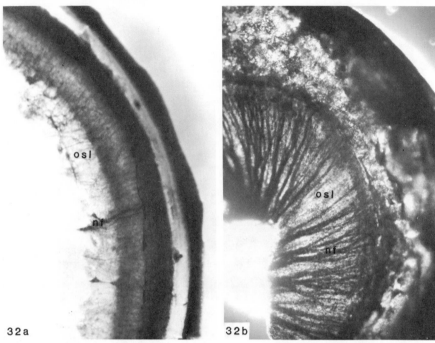

32a   32b

Figure 2-32. Areas from basal (a) and middle (b) turns of the cochlea of a congenitally deaf child. Nerve fiber degeneration appears to proceed from base to apex. An almost complete population of fibers existed in the apical turn even though sensory cells were absent.

exist in the population of approximately 18,000 hair cells.
Outer hair cells are generally more susceptible to damage
than inner hair cells (Figs. 2-29, 2-30), but certainly
there are exceptions to this generalization. Evidence is
accumulating that, in many cases, the actin-containing stereocilia are the structures first affected by acoustic trauma
(Fig. 2-31). As yet this finding has not been investigated
relative to other ototoxic agents. With ototoxic drugs, and
with congenital deafness, organ of Corti damage usually pro-
gresses from basal to apical structure (Figs. 2-30, 2-32);
however, once again, there are exceptions to the generalization. It should be evident that the would be student of
hearing pathology has a multitude of avenues open for
investigation.

Acknowledgments

The technical assistance of R. Mount and the secretarial services of B. Poole are sincerely appreciated. This work was supported by the Medical Research Council of Canada and the Research Institute of The Hospital for Sick Children.

REFERENCES

Babighian, G., Moushegian, G., Rupert, A. and Glorig, A. "Central components of auditory fatigue. Some clinical implications" Proceedings of the Xth World Congress of Otorhinolaryngology, Excerpta Medica 276:95-96, 1973.

Bast, T. and Anson, B.J. The Temporal Bone and the Ear (Springfield: Charles C. Thomas), 1949.

Bredberg, G. "Cellular pattern and nerve supply of the human organ of Corti" Acta Otolaryngologica Supplement 236, 1968.

Fleischer, K. "Untersuchungen zur entwicklung der innenohrfunktion" Z. Laryng. Rhinol. Otolaryngol. 34: 733, 1955.

Lorente de No, R. "Etudes sur l'anatomie et la physiologie du labyrinthe de l'orielle et du VIII:e nerf" Trab. Inst. Cajal Invest Biol. 24:53, 1926.

Trune, D.R. "Influence of neonatal cochlear removal on size and density of cochlear nuclear neurons" Anat. Rec. 190: 566, 1978.

Trune, D.R. "Influence of neonatal cochlear removal on the dendritic morphology of cochlear nuclear neurons" Abstracts of the Fourth Midwinter Research Meeting, Association for Research in Otolaryngology 65, 1981.

Wedenberg, E. "Prenatal tests of hearing" Acta Otolaryngologica Supplement 206, 1965.

Wilson, V.J. and Melvill Jones, G. Mammalian Vestibular Physiology (New York: Plenum Press), 1979.

DEVELOPMENT OF AUDITORY BRAINSTEM RESPONSES

Kurt Hecox
University of Wisconsin, Madison, Wisconsin
Sanford E. Gerber and Maurice I. Mendel
University of California, Santa Barbara

Now we change the topic to electrophysiology and talk about surface recorded electrical potentials. The typical thing is to put a little paste on someone's head, put a metal electrode in the paste, and record the electrical events that ensue following the delivery of signals. What you see depends on when and how you look (Picton et al., 1974). The current way of dividing all of this is according to the time epoch from which you're sampling beginning with the delivery of the stimulus (Fig. 3-1). The so-called cortical evoked potentials are long latency components occurring for several hundred milliseconds and, in fact, for several seconds following the delivery of the stimulus depending on what exactly your stimulus is. Classically one has an inborn P_2-N_2 and those are the landmark points along this time epoch.

If you expand the initial portion, one observes that it is followed by the so-called middle latency components which Mendel discusses in the next chapter. Here again is a sequence of electrical potentials which are easily seen in virtually everyone, and they have their own particular properties functionally in the anatomic generators. Then, if one re-expands this 50 millisecond scale and looks at just the first 10 milliseconds following the delivery of the stimulus, another sequence of waves appears. These waves are the so-called auditory brainstem potentials. We show this only to emphasize again that we are sampling from a very small time epoch of the entire phenomena of the evoked potentials.

Next we try to refine even more the notion of what we are sampling from in order to limit the kinds of conclusions that we can make. Fig. 3-2 is an elegant display (Picton et al., 1974). We focus primarily on Wave I. One feels very firmly that Wave I is the 8th nerve action potential. It is functionally; it behaves exactly like the 8th nerve action potential. Wave II is composed both of secondary discharges of the 8th nerve and early discharges from the cochlear nucleus, primarily the ventral cochlear nucleus. There is no

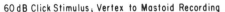

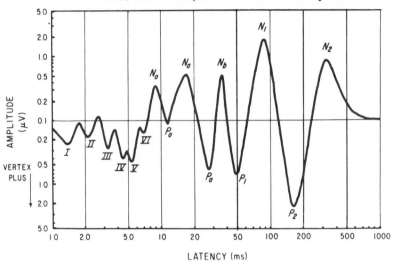

Figure 3-1. Diagrammatic representation of the 15 individual waves of the auditory evoked potentials from eight subjects. Evoked brainstem potentials (1-8 milliseconds) are labeled with Roman numerals (I-VI), middle components (8-50 milliseconds) are labeled N_O-N_b, and the late components (50-500 milliseconds) are labeled P_1-N_2. Latency has been plotted on a logarithmic scale (From Picton et al., 1974).

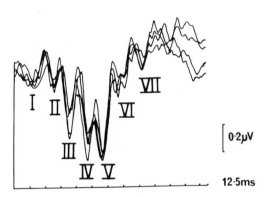

Figure 3-2. Evoked onset brainstem potentials to 60-dB SL clicks presented monaurally at a rate of 1/second. Each tracing represents the average of 1024 responses from vertex-mastoid electrodes. Each latency division represents 1 millisecond (From Picton et al., 1974).

78

contribution from the dorsal cochlear nucleus; none. If you
ablate the dorsal cochlear nucleus, cool it, cut it, burn it,
nothing happens to these recordings. It is in that sense that
we say the dorsal cochlear nucleus makes no contribution.

After that the number of generators contributing to each
of these deflections is multiple. What one can say is that
greater than 60 to 70 percent of the Wave V amplitude (in at
least 3 species) comes from the midbrain region. Now, whether
that is presynaptic or postsynaptic, the relative contributions of lateral lemnisci vs. inferior colliculi neurons is
not well defined. Surely there are superior olivary contributions here too, but they are not statistically as large as
the contribution from midbrain regions.

We have a better idea of generators in this time epoch
than any of the other time epochs. The story is not a simple
one; it is still being worked out. One thing which can be
done is to study pathologic ears, determine what the relationship is between the abnormalities that the patients exhibit on
their audiograms. The brainstem potential is most sensitive
to pathology occurring around the 1000-2000 Hz region. It is
extraordinarily insensitive to any activity below 500 Hz, and
it is very insensitive (and this isn't as well appreciated) to
things at 8000 Hz. Not only is this a poor test of low frequency hearing, it is just about as poor on high frequency
hearing. It is often said that this is a measure of high
frequency hearing, and I think that is inaccurate. We don't
know of anyone who has data showing that 4000 and 8000 Hz are
more accurate than 2000 Hz. The generators for a broad band
stimulus seem to be primarily in the middle frequency range.

Pushing these kinds of comparisons, one finds that the
pathological correlations, in terms of sensitivity measures,
are relatively good. Using data on 200 impaired ears, looking
at the pathologic correlations, 85% of the time one can
exactly categorize the degree of loss. The interest is primarily in the context of identifying people who need to be
pursued vigorously in terms of subsequent evaluation; one can
categorize most people accurately. By using functional
criteria - the properties of the response as you've changed
some stimulus parameter - one can make some determination
about the location of the pathology (Picton, 1978). In Fig.
3-3, for example, the space between the dashed lines represents normal input/output functions, latency vs. intensity
functions; the parallel function occurs in most conductive
pathology. The steep input/output function shown below is

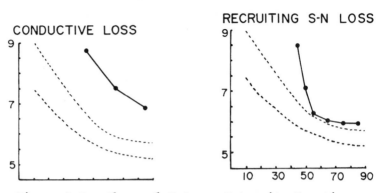

Figure 3-3.   Abnormal Latency-Intensity Functions

seen only in sensory pathology; one can demonstrate that the phenomenon is localized to the inner ear (Picton et al., 1977).

Are these things generated in grey or in white matter? What are the consequences of grey versus white matter in terms of understanding the mechanism underlying auditory development? In Fig. 3-4 are data on patients with multiple sclerosis (Starr and Achor, 1975). There is a prolongation in the amount of time required to go from peripheral nerve to the mid-brain region in these patients who have disordered white matter. We know that, when they improve clinically, as often is the case, their responses may improve clinically; their internodal distances will change. They will decrease internodal distance. We know that there should be increased conduction time because of the decreased conduction velocity that is associated with this reparation process. The auditory brainstem response seems to be quite sensitive to white matter disorders. In fact, one cannot think of a single purely grey matter disorder which results in abnormalities of the brainstem auditory evoked potentials. We don't know whether these are volume conducted action potentials -- i.e., white matter phenomena -- or whether there is some contribution from grey matter graded synaptic kinds of potentials; but the evidence is all indirect, fairly anecdotal, primarily pathologic, that white matter is very sensitive to grey matter pathology. The functional properties, the fact that one can stimulate at 100 or even 115 times per second and still get relatively well preserved responses, argue that most grey matter synaptic kinds of phenomena are not able to do that; most neurons along the

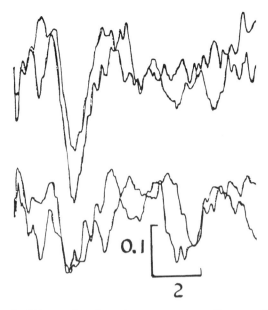

*Figure 3-4. Auditory brain stem response from patient with
multiple sclerosis with clinical involvement of brain stem
structures. Records are in response to monaural click signals
at 75 dB SL. Note that both left-sided and right-sided stimulation evoked wave I of normal latency (1.7 msec) but that the
remainder of records are reduced in amplitude and deviate
substantially from normal (From Starr and Achor, 1975).*

auditory pathway can't do that in terms of the graded potentials. Developmentally, we see, for example, pathologic
instances as maple syrup urine disease or phenylketonuria,
both are associated with abnormal myelin. One would predict,
then, that it would take too long to go from one peak to the
next, and indeed that is the case. Hence, even in developmental white matter disorders, one sees the predicted
phenomena.

What are the kinds of inferences and generalizations we
can make in terms of how the electrophysiology relates to the
behavior that we observe? We have been extremely successful
in pathologic instances primarily because pathology respects
anatomic boundaries and not functional boundaries. It doesn't
mean that, when we're trying to make developmental inferences,
we are going to be as successful. That sort of thing changes
with age.

How do we paramaterize this particular response? The
kinds of things that people look at have to do with the amount
of time between each of the peaks; the interwave intervals.
Primarily one looks at the I-V interwave interval. One also
can look at the relative amplitude of the responses, and the
traditional comparison (primarily because it's a convenient
one) is to compare the amplitude of V to the amplitude of I.
The other thing we can look at is the response to changing
rate of stimulation (Fig. 3-5). The things we initially
looked at are latencies; and, within latencies, absolute
latencies versus interwave latencies; amplitudes, particularly
amplitude ratios; and, then, finally, rate effects.

In Fig. 3-2, we saw the limited amount of variability.
If anything is incredible about this phenomenon, it is the
variability; there is almost none. In adults and in infants,
in the same state, within a session one should get variability
that approaches zero. These responses are highly replicable.
Not as easily appreciated is the fact that wave I is bigger
in newborns than it is in adults (Fig. 3-6), and that accounts
for much of the variability of amplitude ratios. It turns out
that there are really only three waves that are relatively
sturdy: I, III, and V. In fact, we wish we could drop IV and
VI.

Wave I has a time course of maturation in terms of its
latency. In fact, the latency reaches an adult value by about
3 months of age. Waves III and V reach adult values by about
12 months of age (Hecox and Galambos, 1974). We think that's
fairly critical because one of the things we assert is that we
can do essentially an anatomic functional dissection of rates
of maturation. Indeed, the rates of maturation, at least as
reflected by these measures, are not the same for the peripheral auditory system as they are for the central auditory
system. Even when you take into account peripheral anatomic
and physiologic things, there's a lot more to auditory development. But another fairly major message is that one cannot
name almost a single measure that has a time course of maturation beyond about 12 months of age (Fig. 3-7).

One can look at this in even more detail (Fig. 3-8): one
can look at the first through sixth day of life (Cone, 1980).
One can demonstrate developmental phenomena over that very
short period of time, in the first six days of life. One could
have day by day norms, so we take day 3 norms. The I-V latency
changes very little, really, during the first five days. Most
of the first couple of days is a wave one phenomenon. This

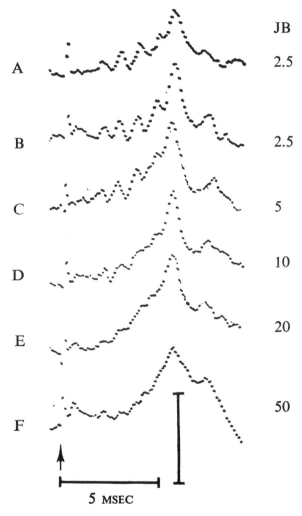

Figure 3-5. Effect of repetition rate on the auditory onset brainstem potentials recorded at the vertex. Numbers at right indicate the repetition rate in stimuli/sec. Click stimulus delivered at the arrow (From Jewett and Williston, 1971).

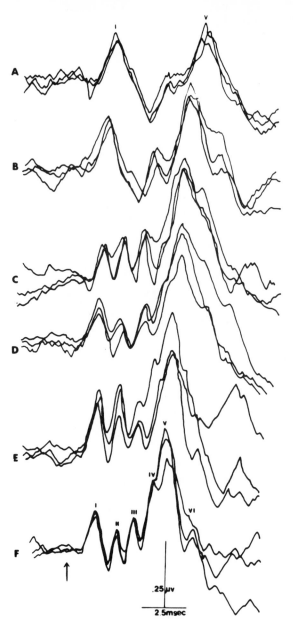

Figure 3-6. Maturational changes in onset brainstem potential waveform as a function of age: A. Newborns. B. Six-week-olds. C. Three-month-olds. D. Six-month-olds. E. One-year-olds. F. Adults. Each trace represents an average of 2400 responses obtained from a different subject. Note also the obvious shifts (shortening) in peak latency with increasing age (From Salamy and McKean, 1976).

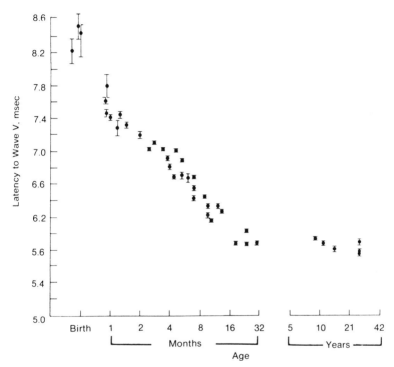

Figure 3-7. Latency of the wave V response to 60-dB SL click as function of age of subject. Systematic decline from birth to 1-2 years is evident. Vertical bars enclose all measurements (at least three) made on given subject (From Hecox and Galambos, 1974).

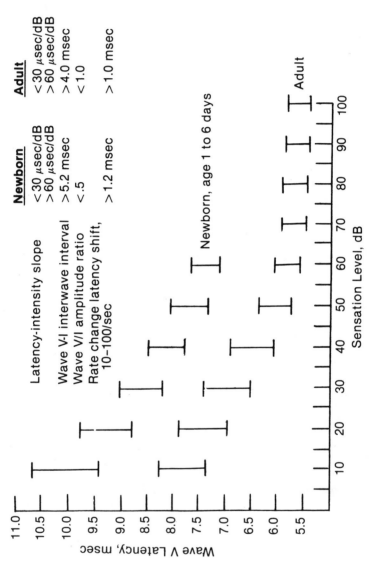

Figure 3-8. Age specific norms for ABR evaluations are necessary for accurate determinations of impairment. Ranges depict mean Wave V latency ± 1 standard deviation. Values for latency intensity slope, Wave V-I interwave interval, Wave V/I amplitude ratio and rate change function indicate those beyond which parameter is abnormal (From Cone, 1980).

probably is a sensitivity change and not something like a
burst of myelin formation or a burst of synaptic transmitter
maturation. It is probably a middle ear phenomenon during
the first 24 hours of life.

In an adult, one looks at these phenomena in a plane by
deciding between which of two electrodes to record. We do
vertical plane by recording from the mastoid to the vertex;
a horizontal plane by recording from mastoid to mastoid. Now,
in an adult, what happens is that, in the horizontal plane,
wave I is very much larger corresponding to the fact that the
dipole of wave I and the dipole of wave V go in different
directions. It turns out, though, that even the orientation
of this electrical phenomenon depends on age. One has to
look at amplitude not just in a single plane but in the dipole space, if one is going to do correlations.

Even after 6 months or 9 months or a year there is still
slight variation in wave I latency. It's a very rapid change
in the first few days, but after this it's very gradual.
We don't know of anybody who demonstrates wave I phenomena
after one year.

One can use tone bursts to do this sort of thing (Picton,
1978). One of the issues, of course, in using a tone burst,
is frequency selectivity. This is a high pass masking phenomenon; you take white noise, high pass filter it, and gradually change the low frequency edge of the high pass noise.
As you eliminate contributions along the basilar membrane
moving apically, at what point do you get a 50% amplitude?
The answer is, for a 400 Hz tone burst, what you get is at
about 600 Hz for the brain stem response. These are both
middle latencies and brain stem responses (Fig. 3-9). About
600 Hz, and at 1600 Hz for the brainstem response, you get a
50% amplitude reduction around 1200 Hz. How tuned are these
responses? If one uses tone bursts one can demonstrate that
they're fairly well tuned, and that one can selectively
stimulate or get maximum stimulation in a region of the
cochlea that matches reasonably well the center frequency of
the signal that you use in normal ears. Frequency selectivity
is very nearly equivalent in adults and neonates with this
measure.

There are data on a patient who has a wave I and nothing
else, and acts behaviorally deaf. Some of these patients
have waves I and III and nothing else. They act behaviorally
deaf (Figs. 3-10A and B). Some patients have I, III, V, and

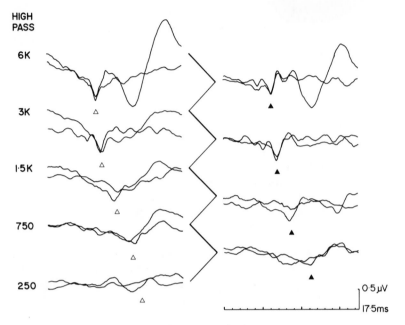

Figure 3-9. The use of high-pass masking techniques to obtain frequency-specific brainstem responses.

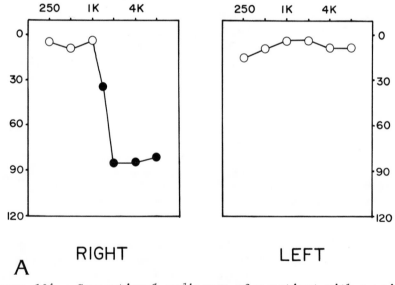

Figure 10A. Conventional audiogram of a patient with a unilateral abrupt high-frequency hearing loss.

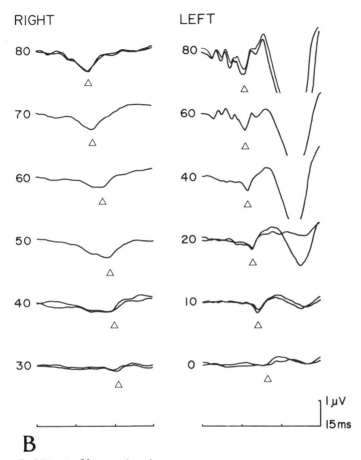

B

Figure 3-10B. Auditory brainstem responses for the patient whose audiogram is illustrated in Figure 3-10A.

no cortical responses; they act behaviorally deaf. The point is that there are lots of ways to get to a single behavioral state. One of the strengths is to describe some of the multiple ways that electrophysiologically one can get to the same behavioral state. Is the problem at the 8th nerve level? Is it the wave V level? Where are differences as a function of age occurring? This extends into the next chapter, which is to say that, when you look at events that are more perceptually oriented, we return to cortical phenomena. This is the world in which perceptual phenomena are going to have their best correlates. While the brainstem response may have

considerable strengths in terms of limited variability, relation to white matter, investigating various phenomena,
traveling wave velocity, etc., many of the perceptual phenomena that one is most interested in are in a whole other time
domain. And that is longer latency phenomena, whether they
are middle or cortical evoked potentials.

REFERENCES

Cone, B.K. "Auditory evoked potentials for pediatric evalua-
    tions" Audiology and Hearing Education 6(3):7-11, 1980.

Hecox, K. and Galambos, R. "Brain stem auditory evoked
    responses in human infants and adults" Archives of
    Otolaryngology 99:30-33, 1974.

Jewett, D.L. and Williston, J.S. "Auditory-evoked far fields
    averaged from the scalp of humans" Brain 94:681-696, 1971.

Picton, T.W. "The strategy of evoked potential audiometry"
    in Gerber, S.E. and Mencher, G.T. (eds.) Early Diagnosis
    of Hearing Loss (New York: Grune & Stratton, Inc.), 1978.

Picton, T.W. et al. "Human auditory evoked potentials. I.
    Evaluation of components" Electroencephalography and
    Clinical Neurophysiology 36:179-190, 1974.

Picton, T.W. et al. "Evoked potential audiometry" Journal
    of Otolaryngology 6:90-119, 1977.

Salamy, A. and McKean, C.M. "Postnatal development of human
    brainstem potentials during the first year of life"
    Electroencephalography and Clinical Neurophysiology
    40:418-426, 1976.

Starr, A. and Achor, J. "Auditory brainstem responses in
    neurological disease" Archives of Neurology 32:761-768,
    1975.

DEVELOPMENT OF PRIMARY CORTICAL AUDITORY RESPONSES

Maurice I. Mendel
University of California, Santa Barbara

In preparing this chapter, I spent time reviewing proceedings so that I could begin with an historical note. One
such publication I reviewed was titled, Conference on Newborn
Hearing Screening, from a meeting held in San Francisco in
1971. I was intrigued by a paper on Neonatal Auditory Testing
presented by my colleague, Dr. Gerber -- both for what it did
as well as did not contain. For example, the section on
"Response Patterns: Electrophysiological" contains an exclu-
sive review of studies carried out on infants with the late
components of the auditory evoked potentials. There is a
brief paragraph describing a so-called "newer technique" --
electrocochleography, first reported as a surgical procedure
by another contributor to this volume, Dr. Ruben and his
colleagues (Bordley, Ruben and Lieberman in 1964). I suppose
my real fascination is with what was not included in that
review only 10 years ago, namely, the topic of the previous
paper, the Auditory Brainstem Response and this paper on the
Middle Latency Responses. From our vantage point in 1982, we
can see that the late components of the auditory evoked potentials receive very little attention these days as a routine
threshold diagnostic procedure, while the auditory brainstem
response appears to be part of the routine audiometric test
battery in many clinics today. If I may be so bold, I would
like to suggest that there even seems to be a resurgence of
interest in primary cortical, or as I prefer to call them,
Middle Latency or Middle Component Responses.

I focus in this chapter on what I think is very appropriately shown schematically in the middle of Fig. 4-1 which
is taken from Picton. I am describing those responses that
occur earlier than the late components, and appropriately for
that reason, are called the middle components, or those events
within the time domain of about 8-50 milliseconds. Hecox, in
the previous chapter, covered a great deal about a number of
very elegant studies that have been carried out in the time
domain of the first 10 or 12 milliseconds. Part of the message
that I would like to impart in my chapter is that there are not

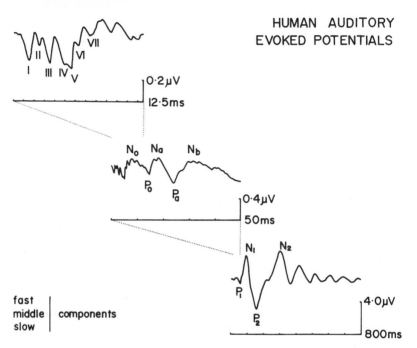

HUMAN AUDITORY
EVOKED POTENTIALS

Figure 4-1. Components of the human auditory evoked potential. Click stimuli of 50 μs. duration and an intensity of 60 dB, S.L. were presented once every second to the right ear. Responses were averaged over 1536 trials from vertex to right mastoid electrodes at three different time bases and three different amplitude calibrations. Negativity at the vertex is shown by an upward deflection. The nomenclature is that of Jewett and Williston for the fast components, Mendel and Goldstein for the middle components, and Davis and Zerlin for the late components (Picton and Smith, 1978).

the number of corresponding studies that I feel there ought to be within this middle latency time domain. I think there are a number of very interesting experimental questions that have yet to be answered about the development of this response and about what this response can tell us about the development of auditory behavior. One of the things that I hope will occur as a result of this book is that we will talk people into pasting on electrodes and taking a look within this time domain.

In this chapter, I do five things with respect to the development of the middle latency responses. I discuss:

1. General parameters of the middle latency responses,

2. Frequency specific information,

3. Origin of the response,

4. Normative studies with infants, and

5. A new reporting scheme for middle latency results.

RECORDING PARAMETERS

Extensive data on recording techniques for the middle
latency responses have been included in at least three
reports (Picton, Woods, Baribeau-Braun, and Healey, 1977;
Mendel, 1977; and Mendel, 1980), so I will not spend time on
these procedures. In general, the recording procedures described briefly in the previous chapter by Hecox also apply to
the middle latency responses. The equipment that is necessary
to record these responses, the electrodes, where we place
them, and how we use them, are essentially the same as used
for the Auditory Brainstem Response. Two notable differences,
however, are the fact that the recording window of the computer is usually set to a 100 msec epoch, and therefore, the
rate of signal presentation must remain below 10 stimuli/sec.
Rates up to 20 stimuli/sec can be used by reducing the recording window to 50 msec. Secondly, the band-pass characteristics of the recording system are usually set to values about
20-100 or 175 Hz. This band of frequencies causes problems
primarily because we are looking within the frequency range
that overlaps the 60 Hz power. Therefore, if the equipment
is not carefully maintained and set up, there are problems
with electrical noise leaking into middle latency responses.
Other parameters - such as electrode configuration, recording
equipment, subject state, etc. - parallel previously described
parameters for the brainstem response.

I will briefly review a sequence of studies that gave us
normative information about the middle component responses
in adults, and move from that into a consideration of frequency
specific information. In one of the early investigations of
the middle component responses, Mendel and Goldstein (1969)
showed that these responses are unchanged as a function of
subject state (Fig. 4-2), which is like the brainstem response
and unlike the later components. No significant differences
were shown in middle component responses with subjects sitting

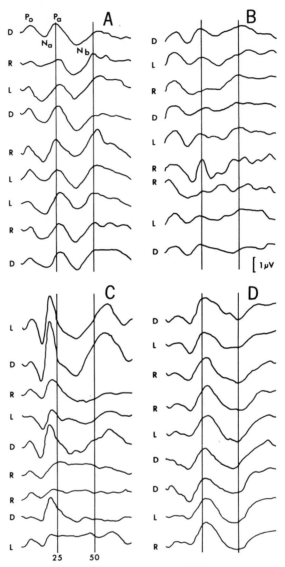

Figure 4-2. Illustrative averaged middle component responses to 1024 clicks at 50 dB SL presented to the right ear at the rate of 9.6/sec. The vertical lines indicate 25 and 50 msec, respectively. Subject A, nine traces very similar; subject B, least consistent of the 12 subjects; subject C, greatest variability in amplitude (note consistent latency); subject D, example of extreme consistency (not included with 22 subjects in data analysis because of slight deviation in sequencing of conditions). D = eyes closed, room darkened; L = eyes opened, room lighted; R = reading (Mendel and Goldstein 1969).

in a lighted room with eyes open, reading under those conditions, or sitting in the dark with eyes closed. Picton and
Hillyard (1974) have shown that the middle components, as well
as the early components, are unaffected by attention, whereas
we can manipulate variables and show the dramatic kinds of
responses that Hecox showed in the previous chapter for the
later components.

Middle components also appear to be unaffected by sleep,
which is a point that I will come back to a little bit later
in my presentation. Fig. 4-3 (Mendel and Goldstein, 1971)
shows a complete night of natural sleep from one subject.
In the awake condition the responses are very similar to those
from the various stages of sleep. The differences that are
apparent in this figure are that, as the subject gets into
deeper sleep at stages 3 and 4, the responses are somewhat
diminished in size. A careful inspection of the figure is
necessary to see the fact that the latency of the major peaks
does move to the right and becomes a bit longer in deeper
sleep. These are shifts on the order of 1 to 2 milliseconds,
so there are minor differences during sleep but these are
relatively minor shifts. Fig. 4-3 shows responses from a
normal hearing adult subject. All of these responses were
obtained with clicks presented at a rate of presentation about
10 per second. Stimuli were presented at 50 dB sensation
level and the clicks were left on for the entire nighttime.
Beginning at approximately 11:00 at night and continuing until
6:30 in the morning, these clicks were presented constantly
to the subject at approximately 10 per second. In stage 2
sleep, for example, at the top of Fig. 4-3 at approximately
11:30 at night until early morning at 6:30 one of the things
that becomes evident is the fact that these responses did not
habituate over time. The fact that there were not dramatic
changes between the different stages of sleep, and the fact
that the responses appeared similar in REM sleep and stage 2
sleep, led us to the realization that we had a stable phenomenon with which to work to investigate the middle component
responses.

The next issue that was attacked with these responses is
the question of audiometric response. How well can we approximate threshold with these responses? In Fig. 4-4, we see percent identification of positive response for the different
stimuli presented. This figure shows that, at 10 dB sensation
level, we were able to identify more than 50% yes responses
for the 4000 and 1000 Hz tone bursts and the click. The 50%
point was identified at the 20 dB sensation level only for the
lowest frequency used, the 250 Hz tone burst.

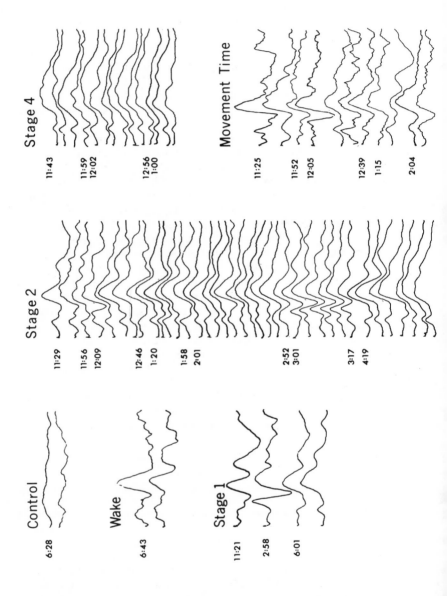

Stage 4

11:43

11:59
12:02

12:56
1:00

Movement Time

11:25

11:52
12:05

12:39

1:15

2:04

Stage 2

11:29

11:56
12:09

12:46
1:20

1:58
2:01

2:52
3:01

3:17
4:19

Control

6:28

Wake

6:43

Stage 1

11:21

2:58

6:01

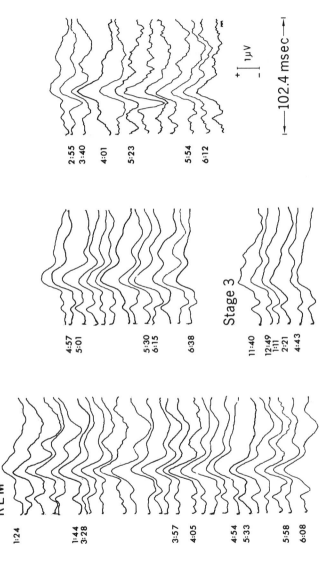

Figure 4-3. All middle component AERs obtained form subject RM for an entire night grouped by stage of sleep and showing representative times of collection. Each trace is an AER to 1024 clicks at 50 dB SL presented at the rate of 9.6/sec. Controls were similarly obtained but without the presentation of clicks. Those AERs spanning a transition from one stage of sleep to another were included with the stage of sleep occupying the greater portion of the time of collection. Movement time encompasses several stages of sleep. Averages were photographically reproduced and are unretouched (Mendel and Goldstein, 1971).

97

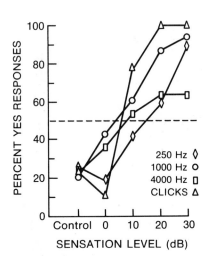

Figure 4-4. Percent of middle component wqveforms judged as meeting predetermined criteria to be considered a response for the different stimuli included in the study. The 50% yes criteria shown by the broken line was defined as the threshold of response identification (Redrawn from Kupperman and Mendel, 1974).

     I'll come back to that issue with respect to the fre-
quency specificity of this response. One of the important
issues is that it is possible to identify these responses at
levels that come fairly close to approximating the adult
behavioral threshold. At the 1981 meeting of the Society for
Ear, Nose, and Throat Advances in Children, there was a session
on the development of auditory behavior in infants. Dr. Wilson
(see Chapter 7) presented a talk in which he refocused on the
issue of identifying responses as an indication of threshold.
One of the points that he made was the fact that, if you go
back into earlier studies, you find that threshold level for
infants is generally approximated at 30-50 dB above our ability
to determine threshold in adults. Over time, as these procedures have become refined and as we have more experience working with these procedures, we found that our ability to predict
threshold in infants comes closer and closer to matching the
adult level. That's not because the infants are beginning to

hear any better, it's because we are becoming a little bit more sophisticated in the use of our various techniques. This holds true in the behavioral domain as well as the electro-physiologic domain. I think that's an important point for us to bear in mind.

The next study on the middle component in adults that was carried out in our laboratory looked at the effect of drugs (Fig. 4-5). We used secobarbitol given in four differ-ent dose levels which were adequate to induce sleep, but none of which was given at anesthetic levels. What we showed was that the middle components appear to be relatively unaffected by the administration of drugs. You see the minimal kinds of shifts that are associated with natural sleep versus the waking state. That is, if you take a particular peak, like P_a, and look at the post-drug state versus the pre-drug state, you see approximately a $1\frac{1}{2}$ to 2 ms shift following the administration of the drug. Clinically, this becomes important to us in that, if we give drugs at levels that are adequate to induce sleep, it helps us to control youngsters who are one and two years old, so that we can carry out our testing technique without wiping out our response paradigm as a function of the administration of the drug. There have been reports (Goff et al., 1977) that anesthetic levels of drugs wipe out middle component responses, but that gets into a different issue.

FREQUENCY SPECIFIC INFORMATION

A major area of importance with the middle components is the frequency specific nature of these responses. Two studies (Thornton, Mendel, and Anderson, 1977; McFarland, Vivion, and Goldstein, 1977) have addressed this issue in adults. Thornton et al. recorded middle components from eleven normal-hearing subjects in response to tone bursts centered at 250, 1000 and 4000 Hz. As shown in Fig. 4-6, amplitude input-output characteristics varied with stimulus frequency and response peak. The most linear input-output characteristics occurred for the early peaks and high stimulus frequencies. However, for routine clinical applications, the extreme frequencies that we chose (250 and 4000 Hz) were too low and too high. In a study published later in 1977, McFarland et al. reported middle components in response to tone pips at 500, 1000, and 3000 Hz. They studied ten normal-hearing subjects and ten subjects with conductive, sensory-neural, or mixed hearing losses. As shown for a normal-hearing subject in Fig. 4-7, similar results were obtained

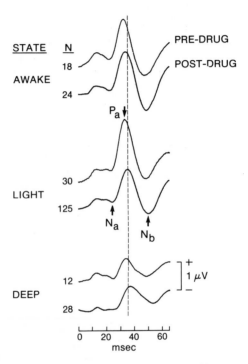

Figure 4-5. Middle components of the auditory evoked potentials as a function of the state from which they were obtained, preceding and following the intravenous administration of secobarbitol. Responses from one subject from the awake, light sleep (stages 2 and REM), and deep sleep (stages 3 and 4) states are shown pre- and post-drug administration. An averaged response consisted of 512 presentations of 1000-Hz tone pips at 40 dB SL at a rate of 9/sec. In this figure, composite responses of the number of individual responses in the N column are shown. For example, the predrug awake waveform includes a total of 9216 (18 x 512) stimuli, while the postdrug awake waveform includes 12,228 (24 x 512) stimuli. (Mendel and Hosick, 1975).

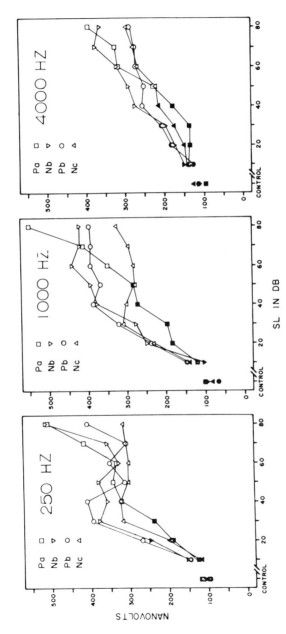

Figure 4-6. Effects of stimulus frequency on the input-output characteristics of four middle evoked potential peaks. Mean peak amplitudes across 11 adult subjects and two trials are plotted as functions of stimulus level. Unfilled symbols are significantly ($p < 0.01$) greater than the control amplitudes (Redrawn from Thornton, Mendel, and Anderson 1977).

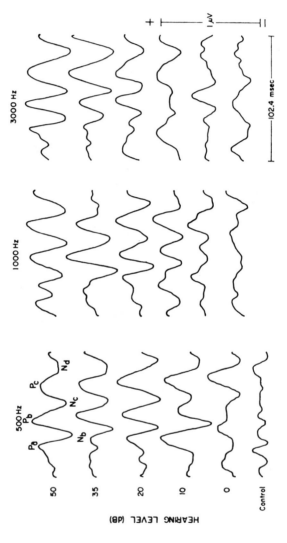

Figure 4-7. Normal-hearing adult subject. Composite middle evoked potentials (N = 1024) as a function of sensation level for three different frequencies. Voluntary behavioral threshold was 0 dB HL for all three frequencies (McFarland et al., 1977).

at each of the three test frequencies, with a small reduction
in latency with increasing stimulus frequency. Notice the
similarity in response pattern at sensation levels as low
as 10 dB. Similar results were obtained from the hearing-
impaired subjects, although latency in this group showed no
clear trend across frequency. However, clear middle components were seen from normal and from hearing-impaired subjects
at all frequencies.

A different procedure for obtaining middle latency
responses to low frequency stimuli was recently proposed by
Galambos, Makeig, and Talmachoff (1981), in which tone pip
stimuli are presented at rates of 40/sec. This response
reportedly disappears with surgical anesthesia, and is
reduced during sleep. This response is also reported at
levels very close to normal adult thresholds.

Voots et al., at a meeting in San Diego in 1976, proposed the use of a compound stimulus to simultaneously
record brainstem and middle component data. As shown in
Fig. 4-8, a click stimulus was followed by a brief period
of time in which to record brainstem responses followed by
the tone burst and then a period of time in which to record
middle component responses. It was interesting that the
inter-signal interval that was chosen appears to be quite
close to this 40 Hz stimulus that Galambos has proposed.
In Fig. 4-9, the first wave is recorded in response to the
click stimulus and the following waves in this particular
response are recorded to the tone burst. This very regular
wave form looks much like the 40 Hz response. In the
bottom of tracing Fig. 4-9 is shown the response to the
click stimulus. This shows that it is possible to record
middle component responses to low frequency stimuli in a
number of different ways, and this is an area that I think
deserves further attention.

ORIGIN OF THE RESPONSE

Although the middle components were the first computer-
averaged evoked potentials to be recorded (Geisler, Frishkopf,
and Rosenblith, 1958), their acceptance into routine clinical
application has long been hampered by the myogenic controversy
first proposed by Bickford, Jacobson, and Cody (1964), as well
as the lack of information relative to the specific site of
origin within the central nervous system (Picton et al.,

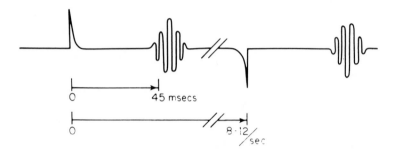

Figure 4-8. Time patterns of compound stimuli are shown with a click at time 0 followed by a 1000 Hz tone burst at 45 msec. Following a variable interval, a second pair of stimuli is presented in the opposite polarity (Voots, Harker and Mendel, 1976).

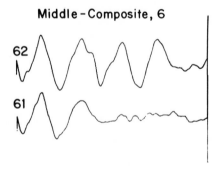

Figure 4-9. Composite middle component responses from six subjects to the compound stimuli shown in Fig. 4-8 presented at 60 dB HL. The lower trace shows the composite response to the click alone (Voots, Harker and Mendel, 1976).

1974). Although myogenic responses can be recorded within
this 8-50 ms time domain at high signal levels or by manipu-
lating electrode position or subject muscle state, I have
long argued that the middle components recorded from relaxed
subjects in response to moderate or low level stimuli are
neural in origin (Mendel, 1977). In a study with Harker
and colleagues at the University of Iowa (Harker et al.,
1977) we recorded middle latency responses to 1000 Hz tone
pips at 50 dB SL during complete muscle paralysis induced
with succinylcholine. We looked at the electromyographic and
middle component activity in the resting state with the subject lying quietly in a sedated state where the subject had
been given valium and a small dose of curare, then totally
paralyzed with succinylcholine, and then allowed to recover.
Fig. 4-10 shows that during succinylcholine paralysis, EMG
activity is totally abolished.

As shown in the right-hand column of Fig. 4-11, similar
middle latency responses were obtained in the resting condition, following sedation, and at the bottom, during skeletal
muscle paralysis. No-stimulus control recordings are shown
during similar conditions in the left-hand column.

While reports of careful research to document the specific
origin of the middle latency responses do not exist, preliminary evidence was presented at the International Electric
Response Audiometry Study Group Symposium in Santa Barbara in
1979 by two groups (Gardi and Bledsoe; and Kaga et al.). The
conflicting results of these two studies further show that
additional research in this area is necessary. I believe the
neurogenic view of the middle latency response to moderate
level signals is commonly accepted. Perhaps one outcome of
this volume will be to stimulate needed research in this
particular area.

NORMATIVE STUDIES WITH INFANTS

But my purpose is not to describe the middle components
from adult subjects. Rather, I will concentrate on development of various measures of middle components in neonates and
infants. There are not many studies in this area, but I
describe below the few that have been reported.

McRandle, Smith, and Goldstein (1974) first reported
repeatable and stable middle components in response to

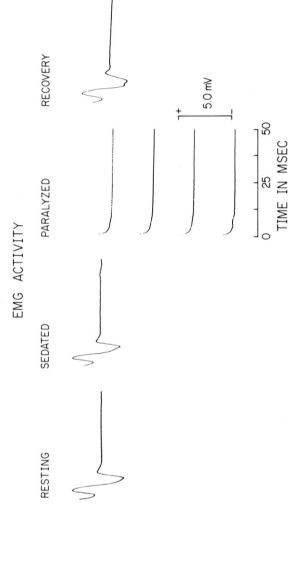

EMG ACTIVITY

RESTING   SEDATED   PARALYZED   RECOVERY

5.0 mV

TIME IN MSEC

0   25   50

Figure 4-10. Photographs of oscilloscope tracings of EMG activity. Normal responses are evident during resting and sedated states and after recovery from skeletal muscle paralysis. No responses are evident immediately before four auditory stimulus presentation sets during paralysis (Harker et al., 1977).

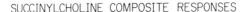

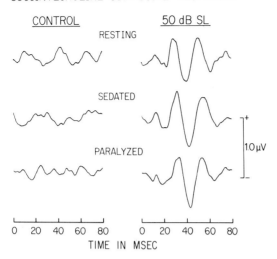

Figure 4-11. Composite responses of 1,600 summed stimulus and control presentations for each test condition showing no clear response pattern in control conditions, and an obvious middle component response in test conditions that appears unchanged during skeletal muscle paralysis. Negative peak at approximate latency of 40 msec is N_b. Positive peaks preceding and following it are P_a and P_b (Harker et al., 1977).

moderate level click stimuli from ten normal newborns, tested 36 to 72 hours after birth. In a follow-up report (Goldstein and McRandle, 1976), 22 additional neonates were studied in a similar manner. The middle component waveforms of all 32 neonates resembled those of adults tested under similar conditions in peak latency and peak-to-peak amplitude. One interesting latency difference was noted: the peak latencies to the 55 dB HL clicks recorded from the left side of the head were shorter than the peak latencies from the right side of the head with left ear signal presentation.

In studies published in 1978 and 1980, Wolf and Goldstein examined middle latency responses in normal neonates. In the first study (1978) tone-pips centered at 1000 Hz were presented at 10, 30, and 50 dB nHL to five neonates. The second study (1980) examined middle components in 20 normal neonates in response to tone pips at 500 and 3000 Hz. Similar results are reported in both studies. The initial portion of the waveforms showed the best agreement with adult responses,

whereas the activity beyond 50-60 ms contributed only minimally to the overall response. The 500 Hz responses (Fig.
4-12) were larger than those at 3000 Hz, and demonstrated
a clearer relation to stimulus magnitude (Fig. 4-13). Unlike
adults', the neonates' middle components were best identified
from the side of the head ipsilateral to the ear stimulated.
These ipsilateral-contralateral differences were further
studied by Reed, Hirsch, and Goldstein, who reported at the
ASLHA convention in 1980. They showed that smaller contralateral responses persisted in babies at least through 28
weeks, but by one year, responses approximated adult
symmetry.

Three studies have been reported on the middle components
in older infants. Horiuchi (1976) studied four infants, aged
12-17 months, with click stimuli and found that the response
pattern was more variable and the peak latencies shorter than
those of adults. Peak amplitudes in infants were smaller
than those of adults, and thresholds for the infants were
approximately 40 dB HL.

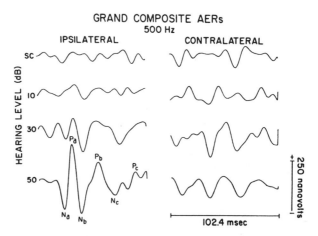

*Figure 4-12. Intensity sequence of the grand composite
middle component averaged electroencephalic response (AER)
waveforms, summed across 10 neonates for the 500 Hz condition. N = 15,360 samples for each AER shown; SC = silent
control (Wolf and Goldstein, 1980).*

In another study, we investigated the middle components
in infants aged one, four, and eight months (Mendel, Adkinson, and Harker, 1977). We presented tone bursts centered at

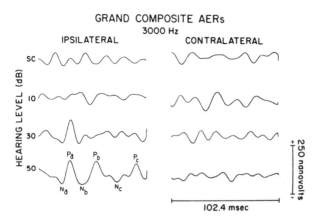

GRAND COMPOSITE AERs
3000 Hz

Figure 4-13. Intensity sequence of the grand composite middle component AER waveforms, summed across same 10 neonates as in Figure 4-12, for the 3000 Hz condition. N = 15,360 samples for each AER shown (Wolf and Goldstein, 1980).

1000 Hz at 15, 30, 45, and 60 dB HL. As shown in Fig. 4-14, similar responses were seen regardless of age. There were no significant differences in latency as a function of age, and only peak P_a showed a significant increase in amplitude as a function of increasing age. As shown in this figure, the amplitude of all three peaks (N_a, P_a, and N_b) showed significant differences as a function of intensity. Responses could be reliably identified at levels of 30 dB and above.

When comparing results from infants to those of adults obtained under similar circumstances (Fig. 4-15), we noted similarities in the first three peaks. Adult subjects tend to show two later peaks, P_b and N_c, which were not usually present in the infants in this study or the neonates studied by Wolf and Goldstein. Like Horiuchi, we found latency values for infants earlier than those of adults, while amplitude values were approximately 200 to 600 nanovolts smaller. In our infant population, we did not find the ipsilateral-contralateral differences noted by Wolf and Goldstein in neonates, however, this is not surprising in view of the fact that our stimuli were presented diotically from a loudspeaker.

In the most recent study, Mendelson and Salamy (1981) recorded middle components from 60 subjects in four age groups - premature infants, full-term newborns, 3 and 4 year olds, and normal adults aged 24 to 39 years. Responses

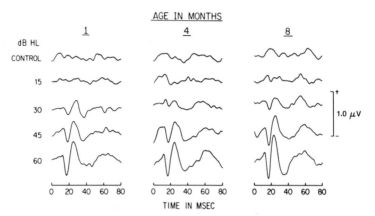

Figure 4-14. Middle component response combined across all six infants at each age and intensity. Tone bursts centered at 1000 Hz were presented during natural sleep (Mendel et al., 1977).

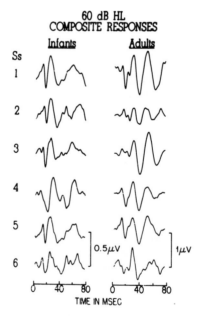

Figure 4-15. Middle component responses from four month old infants and normal hearing adults in response to 60 dB HL stimuli. All subjects were tested during natural sleep (Mendel et al., 1977).

similar in waveform were found in all four groups. Amplitudes of components P_O, P_a, and P_b were found to increase until 3-4 years of age and decline in adulthood. They found no trend for decreasing latency as a function of age, unlike the findings with brainstem and late components (Fig. 4-16). Evidence is presented in this study to show that wave P_O of the middle components is synonymous with wave V of the brainstem response.

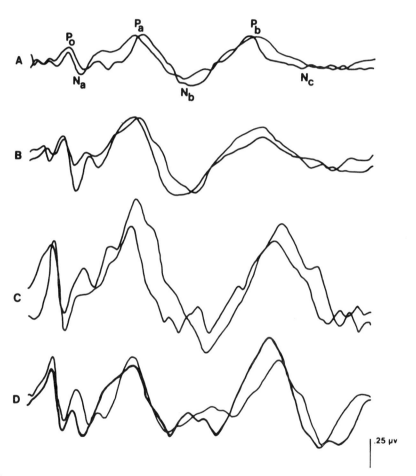

Figure 4-16. Middle component AERs elicited from two subjects in each of the following age groups: A, premature infants; B, full-term newborns; C, 3 - 4-year-old children; D, adults (Mendelson and Salamy, 1981).

RESPONSE REPORTING FORMAT

The final portion of this chapter is devoted to the development of an idea with which I have been grappling for quite some time. It is my contention that clinical acceptance of the middle latency response is impeded by the presentation of too many data in the research reports. Latency data are usually presented for all response peaks, as shown in Fig. 4-17 from Madell and Goldstein. Note the essentially parallel functions for peaks P_o, N_a, P_a, and N_b. One of the factors which I feel has aided the clinical acceptance of the auditory brainstem response is the commonly plotted latency-intensity function of wave V as shown in Fig. 4-18 redrawn from Picton et al. (1977). Many laboratories have replicated these results.

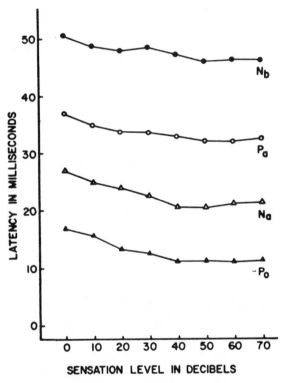

Figure 4-17. Mean latency in milliseconds of four middle component AER peaks for 24 subjects; trials collapsed (Madell and Goldstein, 1972).

Since wave P_a of the middle latency response appears to
be the most robust peak, and is clearly identified in neonates and infants as well as adults, I propose that middle
latency responses be plotted with a similar format. But, I
want to take this argument one step farther. I propose that
the data be shown in a format similar to that of Fig. 4-19,
for peak P_a only, with variability about the mean plotted as
% difference, not in absolute latency. This, I feel, would
lead to a display very similar to that shown in the previous
figure.

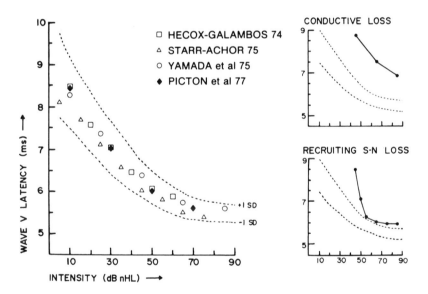

*Figure 4-18. The effect of stimulus intensity on the peak
latency of wave V of the onset brainstem potentials reported
from various laboratories. Wave V latency-intensity curves
are shown for two patients on the right (Modified from Picton
et al., 1977).*

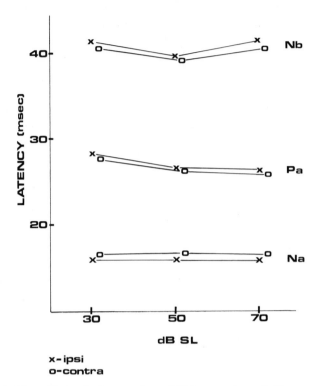

Figure 4-19. Mean latency in milliseconds of three middle
component peaks for 19 subjects; trials collapsed (Mendel
and Sinninger, unpublished).

REFERENCES

Bickford, R., Jacobson, J. and Cody, D. "Nature of averaged
    evoked potentials to sound and other stimuli in man"
    Annals of the New York Academy of Science 112:204-223,
    1964.

Bordley, J., Ruben, R. and Lieberman, A. "Human cochlear
    potentials" Laryngoscope 74:463-479, 1964.

Galambos, R., Makeig, S. and Talmachoff, P. "A 40-Hz audi-
    tory potential recorded from the human scalp" Proceedings
    of the National Academy of Science 78:2643-2647, 1981.

Gardi, J. and Bledsoe, S. "Elucidation of the origins of the middle components (8-25 msec) of the AER in the cat using a serial ablation technique" Paper presented at the Symposium of the International Electric Response Audiometry Study Group, Santa Barbara, 1979.

Geisler, D., Frishkopf, L. and Rosenblith, W. "Extracranial responses to acoustic clicks in man" Science 128:1210-1211, 1958.

Gerber, S.E. "Background paper-Neonatal auditory testing: A review" G.C. Cunningham (ed.) Conference on Newborn Hearing Screening, Berkeley: California Dept. of Health, 1971.

Goff, W., Allison, T., Lyons, W., et al. "Origins of short latency auditory evoked response components in man" in Desmedt, J. (ed.) Auditory Evoked Potentials in Man (Basel: Karger), 1977.

Goldstein, R. and McRandle, C.C. "Middle components of the averaged electroencephalic response to clicks in neonates" in Hirsh, S.K., Eldredge, D.H. and Hirsh, I.J. and Silverman, S.R. (eds.) Hearing and Davis: Essays Honoring Hallowell Davis (St. Louis: Washington University Press), 1976.

Harker, L.A., Hosick, E., Voots, R.J. and Mendel, M.I. "Influence of succinylcholine on middle component auditory evoked potentials" Archives of Otolaryngology 103: 133-137, 1977.

Hecox, K. "Recent advances in the behavioral study of infant audition" in Gerber, S.E. and Mencher, G.T. (ed.) The Development of Auditory Behavior (New York: Grune & Stratton), this volume.

Horiuchi, K. "Auditory middle latency response" Otolaryngology J. Japan 79:1549-1558, 1976.

Jewett, D.L. and Williston, J.S. "Auditory-evoked far fields averaged from the scalp of humans" Brain 94:681-696, 1971.

Kaga, K., Hink, R., Shinoda, Y., and Suzuki, J. "Origin of a middle latency component in cats" Paper presented at the Symposium of the International Electric Response Audiometry Study Group, Santa Barbara, 1979.

Kupperman, G.L. and Mendel, M.I. "Threshold of the early
    components of the averaged electroencephalic response
    determined with tone pips and clicks during drug-induced
    sleep" Audiology 13:379-390, 1974.

Madell, J.R. and Goldstein, R. "Relation between loudness
    and the amplitude of the early components of the aver-
    aged electroencephalic response" Journal of Speech and
    Hearing Research 15:134-141, 1972.

McFarland, W.H., Vivion, M.C. and Goldstein, R. "Middle
    components of the AER to tone-pips in normal-hearing and
    hearing-impaired subjects" Journal of Speech and Hearing
    Research 20:781-798, 1977.

McRandle, C.C., Smith, M.A. and Goldstein, R. "Early aver-
    aged electroencephalic responses to clicks in neonates"
    Annals of Otology, Rhinology and Laryngology 83:695-702,
    1974.

Mendel, M.I., "Electroencephalic tests of hearing" in Gerber,
    S.E. (ed.) Audiometry in Infancy (New York: Grune &
    Stratton), 1977.

Mendel, M.I. "Clinical use of primary cortical responses"
    Audiology 19:1-15, 1980.

Mendel, M.I., Adkinson, C.D. and Harker, L.A. "Middle com-
    ponents of the auditory evoked potentials in infants"
    Annals of Otology, Rhinology and Laryngology 86:293-
    299, 1977.

Mendel, M.I. and Goldstein, R. "The effect of test condi-
    tions on the early components of the averaged electro-
    encephalic response" Journal of Speech and Hearing
    Research 12:344-350, 1969.

Mendel, M.I. and Goldstein, R. "Early components of the
    averaged electroencephalic response to constant level
    clicks during all-night sleep" Journal of Speech and
    Hearing Research 14:829-840, 1971.

Mendel, M.I. and Hosick, E.C. "Effects of secobarbital on
    the early components of the auditory evoked potentials"
    Revue de Laryngologie 96:178-184, 1975.

Mendelson, T. and Salamy, A. "Maturational effects on the
     middle components of the averaged electroencephalic
     response" Journal of Speech and Hearing Research 24:
     140-144, 1981.

Picton, T.W. and Hillyard, S.A.   "Human auditory evoked
     potentials. II. effects of attention" Electroencephalo-
     graphy and Clinical Neurophysiology 36:179-190, 1974.

Picton, T.W., Hillyard, S.A. and Krausz, H.I. et al. "Human
     auditory evoked potentials. I. evaluation of components"
     Electroencephalography and Clinical Neurophysiology 36:
     179-190, 1974.

Picton, T.W., Woods, D. and Baribeau-Braun, J. et al.
     "Evoked potential audiometry" Journal of Otolaryngology
     6:90-119, 1977.

Picton, T.W. and Smith, A. "The practice of evoked potential
     audiometry" Otolaryngologic Clinics of North America 11:
     263-281, 1978.

Reed, N., Hirsch, J. and Goldstein, R.   "Maturation of early
     and middle component AERs in infants" Paper presented at
     the Annual Convention of the American Speech-Language-
     Hearing Association, Detroit, 1980.

Thornton, A., Mendel, M.I. and Anderson, C.   "Effects of
     stimulus frequency and intensity on the middle components
     of the averaged auditory electroencephalic response"
     Journal of Speech and Hearing Research 29:81-94, 1977.

Voots, R.J., Harker, L.A. and Mendel, M.I.   "Three-way ERA
     system simultaneously collects ECochG, early and middle
     responses" Journal of Acoustical Society of America
     60:S16(A), 1976.

Wilson, W.   "Auditory perception" Paper presented at the
     Annual Meeting of the Society for Ear, Nose and Throat
     Advances in Children, Lake Buena Vista, Florida, 1981.

Wilson, W.   "Auditory behavior in infancy" in Gerber, S.E.
     and Mencher, G.T. (eds.) The Development of Auditory
     Behavior (New York: Grune & Stratton), this volume.

Wolf, K.E. and Goldstein, R. "Middle component averaged
    electroencephalic responses to tonal stimuli from normal
    neonates" Archives of Otolaryngology 104:508-513, 1978.

Wolf, K.E. and Goldstein, R. "Middle component AERs from
    neonates to low-level tonal stimuli" Journal of Speech
    and Hearing Research 23:185-201, 1980.

Part II

Behavioral-Perceptual Development

CLINICAL APPRAISAL OF AUDITORY BEHAVIOR IN INFANCY

George T. Mencher
Lenore S. Mencher
Nova Scotia Hearing and Speech Clinic
Halifax, Nova Scotia

This conference focuses on current research in audition: the state of the art. My topic is clinical appraisal, or use of identification and diagnostic techniques; that is, a review of methods which are often years behind research. That is not to say that some clinics are not applying current research. However, in most cases, the same research model applied in the laboratory is rarely, if ever, actively in use in the diagnostic center.

It would be so easy for us in the diagnostic center if we could just hand a child a machine and if he knew what to do to measure his own hearing. Unfortunately, however, most children are just not quite so co-operative. It takes a great deal of organization and a great deal of organized confusion to do a good clinical appraisal of an infant. We have much that we do in a very systematic, organized fashion; and then we have much that we do with that incredible flexibility and spontaneity which allow us to deal with those unusual situations which children create.

The earliest form of clinical appraisal focuses on the newborn or neonate. Several years ago, the United States Joint Committee on Infant Hearing (1972) recommended screening newborns for hearing loss through the use of a "high risk register" or "at risk register". It is not really a register, as children are not registered per se, except, of course, in those states where the program is so structured or mandated by law (e.g., Massachusetts, New Jersey, Arkansas, and Rhode Island). The list of guidelines (the items on the register) includes those factors most likely to cause hearing loss and, thus, the register offers a pool with which the largest number of hard-of-hearing children is likely to be found. Table 5-1 presents the most current (1982) version of the register as promulgated by the Joint Committee.

TABLE 5-1: NEONATAL HIGH RISK REGISTER FOR HEARING LOSS

1)   A family history of childhood hearing impairment.

2)   Congenital perinatal infection (e.g., cytomegalovirus, rubella, Herpes, toxoplasmosis, syphilis).

3)   Anatomic malformations involving the head or neck (e.g., dysmorphic appearance including syndromal and non-syndromal abnormalities, overt or submucous cleft palate, morphologic abnormalities of the pinna).

4)   Birthweight less than 1500 grams.

5)   Hyperbilirubinemia at level exceeding indications for exchange transfusion.

6)   Bacterial meningitis, especially H. influenzae.

7)   Severe asphyxia which may include infants with Apgar scores of 0-3 or who fail to institute spontaneous respiration by 10 minutes and those with hypotonia persisting to 2 hours of age.

In the case of the first item on the list, affected family, we are specifically looking for children whose "blood relatives" have required special schooling, worn hearing aids before age 5, or who have had difficulty in developing normal speech and language due to hearing impairment. If questioning of a parent is not detailed, it is likely that errors will occur and a number of families with individuals with acquired hearing loss (not genetically based) may be included. The resultant confusion and excessive referrals can reflect negatively upon a screening program. Therefore, it is imperative that the parents of children who initially seem to fall on the register because of a family member with a congenital sensory-neural hearing loss be very carefully requestioned before the children are tested or referred. The key is caution to insure that questions concentrate on the total family picture and the presence of degenerative hearing loss anywhere within the entire kinship.

There are, of course, individuals with a delayed onset of hearing loss within the genetic causal category. Sometimes onset occurs within the first or second year, and other times it may not appear until the second or third decade. Thus, even though children with a family history of hearing loss may pass any behavioral screen, they should be followed for the first two years. There is no question that what we know about hereditary, degenerative hearing loss requires that, if a child comes up positive on the register (even if he passes the preliminary hearing screening test), he should be seen again or the family should be contacted again to verify the results.

Guidelines for designating a child as suspect for hearing loss because of severe neonatal asphyxia have been discussed in detail elsewhere (Mencher and Mencher, 1981), and need not be reviewed here. In the course of our study, we have found a few children with no brainstem response but whose parents are absolutely convinced (and we are, too, behaviorally) that they have normal or near normal hearing. Usually at the time of the initial brainstem tests, the child is not responsive to anything. That is, the child has usually failed hearing screening and follow-up in the clinic prior to the brainstem test. It is only after several months that the parents report, "You know, I think so-and-so is beginning to hear". At that time, we do further testing and suddenly we find a child responding behaviorally and sometimes with a brainstem response. What this means is not entirely clear. It does imply, however, that children who are placed on the high risk register because of neonatal asphyxia and who fail hearing screening and follow-up tests initially, may not, in fact, be hearing impaired. There are, of course, implications for other central auditory pathology, but the research is not yet complete on that question. These are things which need to be explored in longitudinal studies. These implications are also true for the meningitis item.

Another item on the "at risk register" refers to congenital rubella or some other perinatal infection. The item concerns what is called the Storch Battery including syphilis, toxoplasmosis, rubella, cytomegalovirus, and Herpes. Clinically, rubella is the best known and, apparently, the most serious of these diseases. However, children who are products of rubella pregnancies are also often the ones who have done the best when you see them several years later. As babies, these infants are the most severely involved, complete with visual, auditory, and cardiac difficulties. At age 10, visual and auditory problems may be well under control; speech and language are often amazingly well developed with speech discrimination much better than expected in view of the audiogram. The few CMV babies we have seen have behaved in a pattern similar to that seen in the rubella

children. That is not surprising in view of the similarity
in the type of damage seen with the two diseases except that
progressive hearing loss has been reported with CMV (Gerber,
Mendel, and Goller, 1979).

Another register item relates to head and neck disorders.
Typically, these are children with cleft palates or those
with anatomical malformations involving the head and neck.
They are quite easily recognizable, and medical treatment is
such that the disorder is usually under good medical and
surgical control. Middle ear disease is frequent in these
children; thus, they need to be followed primarily for that
disorder, as opposed to sensory-neural hearing loss. Of
course, some of the more complex cranio-facial syndromes may
involve cochlear malformations as well, but the majority seem
to be primarily conductive.

Elevated bilirubin level is one of the more controversial
items on the high risk register. The exact level of hyperbilirubinemia which is dangerous to a full term infant and
the best time for measuring that level are both critical
questions. The neonatologist in our center has indicated that
neither 20 nor 25 mg per 100 ml of serum is appropriate. He
indicates it depends upon the actual weight of the child at
the time the examination is done. It is possible to have a
toxic level at 13 or 14 mg, depending upon the weight of the
child. Furthermore, since most such children are treated by
phototherapy before the bilirubin reaches the toxic level,
this item seems to be one which is more academic than real.
Nevertheless, we do consider a child at risk in our center if
he has required an exchange transfusion. There is one sub-
population where hyperbilirubinemia is quite significant,
that being the premature population. These criteria need to
be adjusted according to birth weight. Twenty-five mg per
cent will make most premature children kernicteric. The
problem then may not only be deafness or hearing loss, but
associated CNS sequelae. There should be a guideline for
hyperbilirubinemia which can be recognized and used by lay
persons carrying out a screening program. Until that level
is uniformly accepted throughout the medical community,
"required an exchange transfusion" seems to be a reasonable
alternative.

The item on the high risk register, "Small at Birth",
refers to children less than 1500 gms, regardless of gestation time. This, incidentally, is the only non-etiological
factor on the register. Nevertheless, evidence suggests it

is one of the items most likely to include children with
hearing impairment to any number of causes including middle
ear disease (due to intubation), drug therapy, or actual
disease.

Behavioral Screening

The initial (1970) statement of the Joint Committee did
not recommend mass screening, but urged further studies of
the areas which Gerber has outlined in his chapter in this
text. The second statement, in 1972, recommended the use of
an "at risk register" similar to that just briefly reviewed,
and, further, indicated that children on the register should
be followed in hospitals and clinics. In addition, it was
suggested that a supplemental behavioral test could also be
administered at the time of entry on the register, or shortly
thereafter. The third Joint Committee statement issued this
year (1982) reaffirms the list of high risk items and adds:

> Screening Procedure: The hearing of infants who
> manifest any item on the list of risk criteria
> should be screened under supervision of an
> audiologist, if possible prior to hospital dis-
> charge, preferably by 3 months of age, but not
> later than 6 months of age. The initial screen-
> ing should include the observation of behavioral
> or electrophysiological response to sound. If
> consistent electrophysiological or behavioral
> responses are detected at appropriate sound
> levels, then the screening process wil be con-
> sidered complete except in those cases where
> there is a probability of progressive hearing
> loss, e.g., family history of delayed onset,
> degenerative disease, or intra-uterine infec-
> tion. If results of an initial screening of
> an infant manifesting any at risk criteria are
> equivocal, then the infant should be referred
> for diagnostic testing."

In our nursery, we use three different types of follow-up for
children who are listed on the register. First, we use the
Leridan AudiScreen. The frequency spectrum of that instrument appears as Figure 6-1 in Gerber's chapter in this text.
Based on the spectrum recommended at the Nova Scotia Conference on the Early Identification of Hearing Loss (Mencher,
1976), that instrument has replaced others as the device of
choice for behavioral screening. This has been found

repeatedly and reported by Gerber and Mencher (1979) for full
term neonates and by Gerber (this volume) for pre-term
infants.

The Crib-o-Gram

    The second device utilized for screening in our nursery,
and I would have to say with limited success, is the Crib-o-
Gram (see Fig. 5-1). The Crib-o-Gram is designed to be an
objective method for analyzing the hearing of children. It
consists of a motion sensitive transducer which slips under-
neath the crib mattress. It is responsive to weight between
4 lbs. and 10 lbs. A microprocessor determines that a weight
is present (the baby) on the transducer and that there is no
movement. At this point, the instrument automatically trig-
gers a stimulus presentation through a small speaker. The
transducer will then record any change in movement associated
with the stimulus within a time envelope of about 1½ seconds.
The Crib-o-Gram has three lights located on the left-hand
panel of the machine: 1) a red light - baby has failed; 2) a
yellow light - test still in progress; and 3) a green light -
pass. There are 30 trials given. By relating the probability
of there being no movement on the transducer and then movement
in direct relationship to the stimulus within a time envelope,
the machine uses a statistical probability model to evaluate
each infant: it requires only three definitive responses to
consider the child passed. In spite of the small number, the
mathematical model is quite sound. Most children will not
respond to every trial as they are in deep sleep or habituate
to the stimulus. If the number of non-responses were counted,
most children would be penalized because the machine doesn't
know the child is in deep sleep and is not expected to respond.
The three responses theoretically can happen within the first
three trials. In essence, the instrument requires an outside
envelope of 30 trials, not a stated minimum number of 30
trials.

    One bit of research that could be done with this instru-
ment would be to look at those children who give continuous
responses with every trial or nearly every trial. If a child
continues to respond without adaptation or even when in deep
sleep, it is reasonable to suspect some central nervous
system disorder.

    The Crib-o-Gram has been the source of some mechanical
problems. Its' down time is excessive. The company which
manufactures it now requires every child be tested twice
(within 60 trials), and if the child fails on one of the two

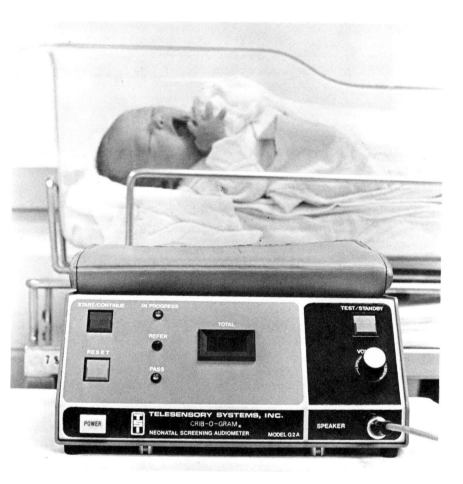

Figure 5-1. The Crib-o-Gram

trials, a third test must be administered. The concept of the unit is excellent, but the mechanism has not yet reached a satisfactory standard.

One major area of some controversy for both the Crib-o-Gram and the behavioral screening is the high sensation level of the test stimulus. Both procedures involve 90 dB SPL. Consider a child with a 70 dB hearing loss with total recruitment by 80 dB. If presented with an 80 dB sound, that child will respond. Thus, children with mild or moderate or low frequency, severe cochlear losses (which include recruitment) may pass the screening. It is true, as some critics indicate,

that the percentage of hearing losses detected with these
methods is highly loaded toward the profoundly deaf and the
high frequency, severely impaired. We are currently investigating procedures for screening at lower intensity levels,
particularly with the Leridan AudiScreen. Because of the
spectrum of that device, we feel that we can utilize lower
intensity levels during testing. Nevertheless, it must be
recalled that the original purpose of these programs was to
identify severely and profoundly impaired and, as the reader
will see later on, we have been successful with that model.
As a bonus, children with middle ear disease have also been
uncovered through these screening procedures.

The key to success is in recognizing the limitations of
these procedures and placing them in a proper perspective.
They are not the only answer or the ultimate answer, they are
the tools we now have available. When early identification
of hearing impairment was a new idea, being able to find a
severe to profound loss at birth was a substantive thing. Our
methods have improved in the clinic and in the experimental
laboratory, so that we are now able to identify some children
with mild or moderate hearing impairments at birth. This was
relatively unheard of 15 years ago. As our laboratory techniques improve and reach clinical application, I feel relatively comfortable in stating, we will be applying them,
either by reducing the intensity level of our screening procedures or changing and refining our techniques with increased
success. Nevertheless, what the future holds does not negate
what we are able to accomplish with our current procedures.
It is a classic example of research and clinical effort being
in two separate time domains. There is no question that
electrophysiological methods can and do provide a more
detailed, and therefore I suppose, a better view of a child's
auditory sensitivity. However, clinically, these techniques
usually take hours, cost many dollars, and require very
sophisticated equipment and highly trained personnel. Is
that screening? No. Therefore, until research can provide
cheaper, faster, and more accurate means of screening than
the AudiScreen or the Crib-o-Gram, we must be willing to
screen at somewhat higher levels and to look only for the deaf
and profoundly hearing impaired, and not be so critical of
those techniques which we can utilize. As a clinician I say,
"When a procedure has been developed which, for $1.00 or $1.25
per child, can identify the mild to moderate hearing impaired,
as we now can with the profoundly impaired or the deaf, we
will welcome with open arms the adoption of that procedure."
Furthermore, that procedure must be applicable not only in the

major medical centers throughout the world, but also should
be applicable in "Podunk Hospital, Small Town, U.S.A." Therefore, it seems criticism of current techniques is correct,
but highly inappropriate in terms of current, realistic,
clinical appraisal, available equipment, money, and personnel.

There could be a question raised as to whether mass
screening is providing parents with misinformation. That is,
it is giving families a sense that their babies have normal
hearing without the parents realizing that the children have
been screened at a very high level of sound. That is a valid
criticism and an important reason for insuring that every
child is screened in complete compliance with the recommenda-
tions of the Joint Committee, and is followed during infancy.

The Infant Hearing Assessment Foundation

Recently, in an effort to blend laboratory effort while
trying to overcome high cost objections, a "brainstem" screening program has recently come on the scene. Called Infant
Hearing Assessment Foundation, it operates what is called the
IHAP or Infant Hearing Assessment Program. Funded primarily
by the Telephone Pioneers of America, the foundation produces
a brainstem screening device called "Synap I" (see Figure
5-2). The program is run entirely by volunteers who are under
the supervision of an audiologist. The instrument is pro-
grammable in that the number of clicks being presented to the
infant and the intensity levels at which they are being presented can be altered. The intensity range is from about 70
dB to 25 dB SPL. Scoring is based on a very simple premise.
The examiner is asked to indicate the presence or absence of
Wave V. There is no concern regarding Wave V latency, amplitude factors, or interpeak latency. The purpose of the
machine is merely screening hearing by indicating the presence or absence of a Wave V at two different test levels.
The child would be scored a pass if a Wave V is present at
both levels. In our nursery we have been using the Synap at
approximately 55 dB HL and 35 dB HL for screening. We are
using it only in the intensive care nursery.

There has been some controversy about this machine and
the Pioneer program. Controversy surrounds the general program first, because the system has been developed by the
Pioneers for use with volunteers in the intensive care nursery. Volunteers are usually not welcomed en masse in that
environment. A second area of controversy concerns the sound

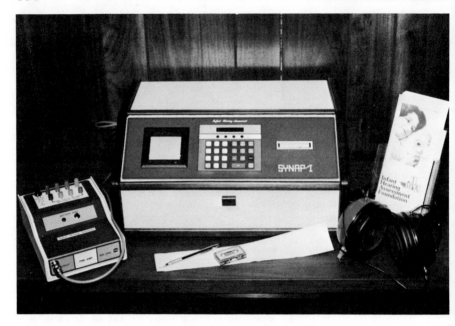

Figure 5-2. The Synap-I

level standards utilized on the machine itself. A third area
concerns the absence of an artifact reject as an integral part
of the instrument.

The principle of applying some sort of brainstem screening in the neonatal unit, nevertheless, is the major principle
we are discussing. Table 5-2 illustrates the mean latency
times for Wave V for babies seen in our center, compared to
established norms (Harris et al., 1981; Cox et al., 1981).
It is apparent that our norms with the Synap I are well within
other norms published in the literature.

The question of volunteers has been a major issue for us.
First of all, our neonatology department does not welcome
large numbers of them in the Intensive Care Unit. Secondly,
many of the volunteers are skeptical about their own capacities in such a setting. They are afraid of hurting the child
or being "underfoot". Some are also intimidated by the hustle
and bustle of a large medical situation. On the other hand,
we have found one or two individuals who are so well self-
disciplined, interested, and willing, that they have made the
entire Synap I program successful. We have learned in our
center that the volunteer program can work, if:

Table 5-2: LATENCY TIME FOR WAVE V

Gestational Age in weeks	Harris et al. 50 dB HL	Mencher (Synap) 54 dB HL	Cox, Hack, and Metz 60 dB HL
35 - 36	7.49	7.34	7.85
N	(4)	(11)	(22)
37 - 38	7.09	7.24	7.79
N	(24)	(20)	(20)
39 - 40	7.03	7.23	7.65
N	(52)	(18)	(14)
41 - 42	6.95	7.05	
N	(35)	(42)	

131

1) volunteers are carefully screened and appropriately chosen;

2) only a limited number is chosen;

3) volunteers are under direct supervision;

4) they are individually trained.

We are very proud of those people who help us in our Synap
program, and feel that the Telephone Pioneers have made a
significant contribution these past few years.

The controversy concerning a lack of an artifact reject
built into the Synap I is less of an issue to those of us
who use the instrument than those who criticize it from a
theoretical point of view. Our staff (both professional and
volunteer) have learned how and when to put the unit on "hold"
when an artifact is present. Our information, for screening
purposes, is accurate and is not adversely affected by the
lack of an artifact reject. It is true that an artifact reject would be essential if we used the Synap I for clinical
diagnostic purposes. However, it is not a major factor when
screening is the primary function, as is the case with the
Synap machine. It must be recalled that that machine was
developed solely for the purpose of screening.

Test time is long, an average of 45 to 60 minutes per
child. That is too long for a screening program. Cost is
low, but that is because of the generosity of the Telephone
Pioneers of America and the efforts of a non-paid volunteer
staff. With time and cost controls, the program is quite
viable. Without them, I believe, use of ABR instrumentation
would be far too costly, far too time consuming, and frankly,
really, an "overkill" when we are trying only to screen a
child's hearing. I have no doubt that those parameters will
change within the next two to three years, and ABR screening
will become the modus operandi.

Results of the Nova Scotia Newborn Screening Program

Over the last 40 months, utilizing the high risk register
and behavioral screening, we have examined more than 16,000
children born in the Halifax, Nova Scotia, area. Table 5-3
illustrates the data from that project. The SNCU data refer
to children who were in the intensive care unit but not on
the high risk register. The children up for adoption were
also screened in a sub-project. None of those children failed.

TABLE 5-3: GENERAL STATISTICS - NOVA SCOTIA HEARING AND
     SPEECH CLINIC NEWBORN HEARING SCREENING PROGRAM
                (January, 1978 - April, 1981)

Number of Months: 40

Number of Births: 16,312

    1) High Risk   -   2222

    2) SNCU   -   1397

    3) Adoption   -   421

    4) Mother's Request   -   994

    5) Miscellaneous   -   652
                                    _____

                   TOTAL TESTED   5686

Number Failed: 293 (1.8% of those born; 5.2% of those
                behaviorally screened)

We are now no longer automatically screening children being
considered for adoption, unless we are requested to do so by
the adoption agency.

    Our general program included a behavioral follow-up of
5,686 children. Of those 5,686 children, 293 failed the
behavioral screen by the AudiScreen or equivalent procedure.
That means we failed 1.8% of those born, or 5.2% of those
screened.

    Table 5-4 illustrates the high risk categories of those
with confirmed hearing losses. These include conductive
hearing losses as well as sensory-neural. The majority of the
sensory-neural losses are in the small at birth group and the
neonatal asphyxia category. The other categories are primarily conductive, except, of course, those from affected
families. One interesting thing is that we have three children
in the SNCU with a confirmed hearing loss who are not on the
high risk register. On the basis of those data, we have modified the high risk register from the list seen as Table 5-1.
First, bacterial meningitis was added. This was done on the

TABLE 5-4:   HIGH RISK REGISTER STATISTICS - NOVA SCOTIA
HEARING AND SPEECH CLINIC HEARING SCREENING PROGRAM

Number Failed			Confirmed Hearing Loss
Asphyxia	=	64	2
Bacterial meningitis	=	32	4
Congenital rubella or other virus	=	0	0
Defects of head or neck	=	17	1
Elevated bilirubin	=	1	0
Stay in neonatal intensive care unit 5 days	=	23	9

SNCU = 81

Adoption = 27

Mother's Request = 31

Miscellaneous = 21

          N = 293   N = 19

recommendation of the Joint Committee and follows on the basis
of our own information.   Secondly, instead of "small at birth",
as on the original register, we changed the register to "stay
in the neonatal intensive care unit for greater than five
days".   Obviously that category includes those children who
are small at birth and were not on the high risk register.
It should be pointed out, again, that a stay in the intensive
care unit for five days is not a cause or etiological factor
for hearing loss.   However, most of the categories do overlap
with this one, so the category offers redundancy.   We believe
this is a healthy part of the screening procedure.

Once a baby has failed the newborn screening, we transfer
the child to the audiology center where we look "clinically"
at reflex and/or startle behavior.   For older children, we
try conditioned orientation reflex techniques which include
the visual reinforcement audiometry procedures in Chapter 7.

Clinical Behavioral Testing

What is commonly called the Ewing Method, involving head turn and localization, seems to be very helpful in working with these children (Northern and Downs, 1978). Wilson and Gerber, in Chapter 7, suggested that this work may be predicated on some earlier ideas of Murphy in England. He has also suggested that it may not have a scientific basis in real behavior. While he is most likely correct, the methodology and guidelines do appear to work in our clinic.

The psychologists, notably Muir and Field (1979), have provided information regarding the behavior of children below four months of age, which may be far more accurate than the protocols listed by Northern and Downs. However, because of the restricted time envelope (within one or two seconds) utilized in most clinical approaches compared to the time envelope (10 to 15 seconds) allowed in most psychological developmental normative studies, the apparent contradiction between results does not seem to have diagnostic application. Northern and Downs (1974) may be marginally incorrect in their statements about the localization skills and behavior of children under four months of age, but the clinical behavior we see in the diagnostic situation supports their claims for most children. Perhaps it is necessary for audiologists to modify clinical approaches to allow for the developmental data the psychologists have been providing for us. But until then, it is another case of research-laboratory effort not yet blossoming into clinical application.

Impedance

Impedance is another clinical technique which is very difficult with babies. We have found it to be an almost useless technique with the newborn because: 1) the ear canal is so small the probe will not fit in properly; 2) the children are not really cooperative; and 3) often the tympanograms will actually reflect movement of the ear canal and not movement of the tympanic membrane. We have tried using the new automatic tympanometers with a little better success, but the ear canal of most infants is so tiny that we have not found the device to be useful. It is recommended that, when impedance is done with a baby, the child should be in a sitting position. If the head is in a flat position, it may change the position of any fluid in the ear and result in a normal tympanogram in the presence of middle ear disease.

The importance of impedance should not be overlooked in spite of the difficulties in administering the procedure. Downs (1981) reviewed data at a U.S. Joint Committee meeting in which she discussed otitis prone infants. In both a retrospective study and an ongoing study, she reported the incidence of middle ear disease in children was significantly higher for children who had initially resided in a neonatal ICU. It is easy to see how the high number of otitis prone newborns can be present in the ICU, as these children are primarily in a lying position and often have been through some form of intubation.

Summary

The conclusion one can draw from these preceding pages is simply that it is possible to identify a group of children at birth who are at risk for hearing impairment. It is difficult to follow those children, but not impossible. As a result of good conscientious clinical efforts, it is possible to identify deafness in the newborn. Finally, experimental research is providing us with newer and more advanced methods which will make our search that much easier to carry out and which will enable us to travel that rather rocky path with a surer foot.

REFERENCES

Cox, C., Hack, M., and Metz, D. "Brainstem-evoked response audiometry: normative data from the preterm infant" Audiology 20, 53-64, 1981.

Downs, M.P. personal communication, 1981.

Gerber, S.E. and Mencher, G.T. "Arousal response of neonates to wide band and narrow band noise" Paper presented at the annual convention of the American Speech-Language-Hearing Association, Atlanta, Georgia, 1979.

Gerber, S.E., Mendel, M.I., and Goller, M. "Progressive hearing loss subsequent to congenital cytomegalovirus infection" Human Communication, 4, 232-233, 1979.

Harris, S. and Almqvist, B. "ABR in operatively verified cerebello-pontine angle tumors" Scandinavian Symposium on Brain Stem Response, Scandinavian Audiology Supplement 13, 113-114, 1981.

Joint Committee on Infant Hearing Screening Statement of
    November 1970, Asha 13, 79, 1971.

Joint Committee on Infant Hearing Screening "Supplementary
    statement, July 1, 1972" Asha 16, 160, 1974.

Joint Committee on Infant Hearing "Position Statement, 1982"
    Pediatrics. 70(3), 496-497, 1982.

Mencher, G.T. (ed.) Early Identification of Hearing Loss
    (S. Karger: Basel), 1976.

Mencher, G.T. and Mencher, L.S. "Auditory pathologies in
    infancy" Paper presented at the Conference on Auditory
    Development in Infancy, Erindale symposium, Ontario,
    Canada, 1981.

Muir, D. and Field, J. "Newborn infants orient to sounds,"
    Child Development 50, 431-436, 1979.

Northern, J.L. and Downs, M.P. Hearing in Children, second
    edition. (The Williams & Wilkins Company: Baltimore),
    1978.

Wilson, W.R. and Gerber, S.E. "Auditory behavior in infancy"
    In The Development of Auditory Behavior, Gerber, S.E.
    and Mencher, G.T. (eds.), this volume.

AUDITORY BEHAVIOR IN THE NEONATAL PERIOD

Sanford E. Gerber
University of California, Santa Barbara

When examining the behavior of newborns in response to acoustic events, it is necessary to ask a number of rather specific questions. These questions deal with "stimuli, response patterns, environmental factors, and behavior of observers" (Gerber, 1971). This chapter is primarily concerned with only one of those questions: "Which acoustic events serve as the best stimuli for infants?" Even to raise a question regarding stimuli implies that we know a good deal about what constitutes a response. Evidence suggests that we do (Taylor and Mencher, 1972; Mencher et al., 1973).

The majority of the time what constitutes a response prenatally is not the same as what we are willing to accept as a response postnatally. The main studies of prenatal audition are those of Johansson et al. (1964) and of Tanaka and Arayama (1969). In general, these investigators observed that the human fetus will respond to acoustic stimulation by some change of motor activity -- which might be attested to by any mother -- and by a change of cardiovascular rate. These two kinds of responses are equally as valid post-natally as they are prenatally. Fortunately, however, we have better and less complicated ways of assessing post-natal response behavior.

A large and confusing variety of observable behaviors has been taken as indicators of neonates' responses to sound. These include (inter alia) changes of position, alterations of apparent respiratory activity, crying, assorted eye movements or limb movements, and immobilization. In fact, it was this confusing array of behaviors which supposedly would satisfy response criteria, but which really did not, that led the Nova Scotia Conference on Early Identification of Hearing Loss (Mencher, 1976) to lay down a specific and narrowly defined set of behaviors to describe a neonate's response to sound. Called an "arousal response", it is defined as "any generalized body movement which involves more than one limb and which is accompanied by some form of eye movement."

Furthermore, the Nova Scotia Conference required that these simultaneous behaviors must be reported by two independent observers on a minimum of two of eight trials. For purposes of this discussion of stimulus properties, and in accordance with studies of neonates' responses in behavioral screening programs, a response is defined as that set of motor behaviors prescribed by the Nova Scotia Conference.

The general question of stimulus properties, as it turns out, has to do with bandwidth. Studies of narrow band signals have shown them to be most unsatisfactory stimuli. Mendel (1968) observed that four- to eight-month-old infants gave more responses to broad band signals than to narrow band noise or to warble tones. Bench (1969) compared 85 dB signals of 500 and 2000 Hz and found that there were no significant differences in the response-eliciting properties of these two tones. In a subsequent study, Bench and Mentz (1975) determined that tonal stimuli are "very inefficient as regards eliciting responses." Similarly, Gerber et al. (1976) found no difference between a narrow band noise centered at 3000 Hz and a tone which is frequency modulated around 3000 Hz. In other words, given equal spectral density over a narrow bandwidth, spectral details are not important. But, Ling et al. (1970) found a 1/3-octave band centered at 2000 Hz to elicit more responses than one at 3150 Hz and also more than a sine wave signal. They did not use wider bands. In fact, one serious problem has been the ineffectiveness of these stimuli to discriminate hearing-impaired from normal hearing infants (Hardy et al., 1970).

Furthermore, narrow band signals seem to not work very well. It appears, in fact, that only one researcher has found narrow band signals to be satisfactory. Her data, however, are curious indeed. Franklin (1980) claims that she "has successfully applied narrow speech bands to determine hearing thresholds for numerous infants, children, and retarded and deaf-blind adults..." But the paper in which she makes this claim reports on only 18 subjects ranging in age from 2 months to 37 years. It may be that narrow bands of speech serve as satisfactory stimuli for deaf, blind, and/or retarded persons who are 37 years of age, but all the other evidence is that narrow band signals are not effective for children under the age of one month. More recently, she has observed no differences among several narrow bands which were presented to neonates (Franklin, 1981).

Bench and Mentz (1975) proposed that defining stimulus complexity in terms of frequency bandwidth is "of major importance" when eliciting behavioral responses from infants. In 1972, Taylor and Mencher had observed that white noise elicited the largest number of responses from their large sample (225) of infants, but also observed that children with "corner" audiograms might respond to white noise. Bench et al. (1976) determined that use of a broad spectrum noise (as compared to narrow band noise or speech) increased the probability of eliciting an unconditioned behavioral response from a neonate. Therefore, given that wide band stimuli do seem to be better response elicitors than narrow band stimuli and given that, as clinicians, we wish to avoid false positive responses among children who have corner audiograms, the Nova Scotia Conference recommended a signal that would meet these objections. The "Nova Scotia Spectrum" is essentially high-pass-filtered white noise. It is a broadband signal which falls off at the rate of 30 dB per octave below about 750 Hz (Figure 6-1). However, it was not until 1979 that this spectrum was actually compared with the narrow band signals (frequency modulated tones or narrow band noises) generated by commercially available devices.

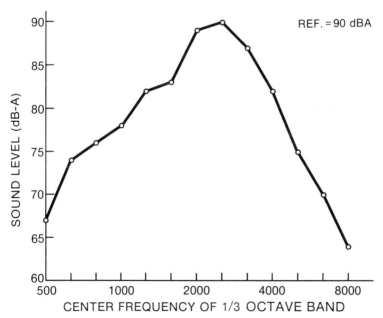

Figure 6-1. The Nova Scotia Spectrum

Gerber and Mencher (1979) compared the Nova Scotia
Spectrum to a narrow band noise which peaked at 3000 Hz
(Figure 6-2). The paradigm for this experiment was that
each infant received eight bursts of each signal with an
interstimulus interval of 15 seconds in a counterbalanced
procedure. The counterbalancing was accomplished by having
half the infants receive eight narrow band signals followed
by eight wide band signals, and the other half receive eight
wide band signals followed by eight narrow band signals.
There were two important findings from this study on 47
children in the first few days of life. The first was that
the wide band noise elicited more responses than the narrow
band noise from virtually every infant. The second important
finding was that the wide band signal seemed to be more
attention-getting, if we define that by noting on which signal presentation the infant first responds. Generally,
infants respond sooner to wide band than to narrow band
signals.

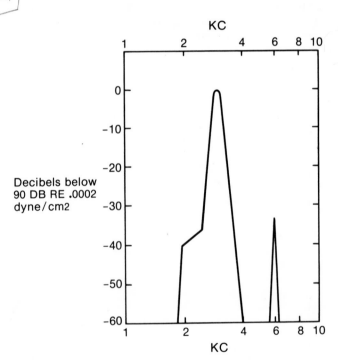

Figure 6-2. The Narrow Band Spectrum

Why should infants in the first few days of life be more responsive to wide band signals than to narrow band signals? Although the issue of stimulus complexity has been discussed repeatedly by Bench and also by Eisenberg (1969), there may be another parameter at work. Loudness increases with bandwidth at least up to a critical band and probably up to bandwidths as great as one octave. Hence, although we cannot directly measure loudness responses of neonates, we know that a wide band signal of a given sound pressure level is louder than a narrow band signal at the same sound pressure level. Hence, it may be that the infants' apparently increased responsivity to wide band signals is, in fact, responsivity to greater loudness.

To answer this question, Mason (1981) played the same two signals employed by Gerber and Mencher (1979) to a listening panel of adults who equated the signals for loudness in a customary AB matching experiment in which the loudness of the narrow band signal was fixed at 90 dBA. Results indicated that the wide band signal needed to be about 3 dB less intense than the narrow band signal in order to be perceived as equally loud. Then, as part of the same study, a 90 dBA narrow band signal and an 87 dBA wide band signal were presented to 22 normal full-term, newborn infants. The results again showed that infants were more responsive to the wide band signal than to the narrow band signal.

Stimulus complexity (i.e., bandwidth) was found to exert a differential effect on the frequency of neonates' arousal to acoustic stimulation. Mason's results indicate that the Nova Scotia spectrum was more effective at eliciting arousal responses from normal newborns than an equally loud narrow band stimulus (3000 Hz frequency modulated tone). While a response bias toward the wide band over the narrow band stimulus was expected, even with loudness controlled, what was unexpected was the magnitude of the obtained differences in response rate across these stimuli. Mason observed that, 'since the wide band stimulus is inherently louder than the narrow band due to energy over a wider range of frequencies," the possibility existed that at least part of this difference in response eliciting effectiveness was due to the difference in loudness as well as differences in bandwidth. With the loudness advantage of the wide band signal removed, it was anticipated that the wide band signal would continue to evoke more responses than the narrow band but not that it would elicit proportionately even more responses than when it was perceptually louder." Mason's study found that the wide

band signal elicited more than two-thirds more responses than
the narrow band signal, notwithstanding their loudness
equivalence.

Moreover, the wide band stimulus evoked not only more
responses, but responses from more and younger neonates.
Among infants who responded to only one of the two test
signals, the overwhelming majority (10/11) was aroused by
the wide but not the narrow spectrum signal. Even children
under the age of 24 hours (who are relatively unresponsive
to hearing screening signals) were observed to give clear,
easily discernible arousal responses to the wide band signal
on 80% of the trials. In contrast, seven of the 10 neonates
under 24 hours did not respond at all to the narrow band
signal. Furthermore, not only were there more responses to
wide band (87 dB) than to narrow band (90 dB signals), they
occurred sooner in the series.

The Mason (1981) study has now been replicated using
pre-term infants. In this investigation (Gerber et al., in
press), we again observed the same large difference between
the arousing properties of the two spectra. Furthermore, it
was shown that pre-term infants were more responsive than the
full term infants employed by Gerber and Mencher (1979) or
those used by Mason. It seems, therefore, that the notions
of Bench and Eisenberg about bandwidth as stimulus complexity
are indeed valid independent of gestational age.

There is an ongoing desire to employ signals of less
intensity for screening purposes (Chapter 5). Historically,
most investigators and clinicians have used 90 dB signals
to screen hearing among neonates. What has been screened
by using such an intense signal is the profoundly hearing
impaired from all others. Of course, that is desirable, but
it would be still better if it were possible to also screen
out even those with moderate impairments.

Where do we go from here, then? The answer to this
question is the same as the resolution of the issue just
raised. It would be important and interesting to know at
what intensity levels wide band and narrow band signals are
equal in their ability to get responses. This not only provides a measure, however indirect, of the effect of loudness
and of stimulus complexity, it also might teach us at what
level we could be screening neonates with wide band signals.
Furthermore, since wide band signals seem to get responses
sooner than narrow band signals, we want to investigate this

uestion as well. For this observation, by the way, I am
ndebted to my colleague Dr. Mendel. He noted that increasing
he interstimulus interval might have a perceptual effect of
aking each stimulus novel. One theory of perception (Broad-
ent, 1958) posits that a signal must be novel to elicit a
esponse. It is a cause of continuing concern that, clini-
ally, we accept two responses out of eight trials as passing
Gerber et al., 1977) indicating that we are willing to accept
nly 25% correct as good enough. This is, of course, a le-
itimate procedure according to statistical analysis and the
se of probability theory (Mencher et al., 1973). Hence, if
e can get responses to the first stimulus presented, then
t might be possible to increase the interstimulus interval
o such a time that every signal presentation is, in effect,
first stimulus.

Of course, clinically we don't give the child eight
rials unless he is failing: if he responds to the first two,
e stop testing. What we report here is an experimental
aradigm, not a clinical one. In the experimental paradigm,
ach infant receives sixteen stimulus presentations. It is
mprobable that sixteen signal presentations would be used
n a clinical assessment. The standards of the Nova Scotia
onference, adopted by the Joint Committee on Infant Hearing,
onsider a positive response to be two out of eight trials.
learly, then, if the infant responds on, say, two of the
irst three trials, the remaining five presentations are not
iven. Therefore, in a clinical paradigm, results such as
hese may not be found. Let us suppose, for example, that a
iven infant responds four times on eight trials to the wide
and signal but responds only twice out of eight trials to
he narrow band signal. If we require only two out of eight,
nd we stop testing when we get two responses, we could easily
e unaware that the wide band signal is a better response
licitor. The effect of this, then, is to urge the clinician
o use the wide band signal and thereby increase the proba-
ility that a normal hearing infant will respond on the first
ew trials.

The conclusion, then, is obvious. We have at least these
wo studies to do soon: one on increased loudness differences
nd one on increased interstimulus intervals. I think, too,
hat we want to look at wide band signals which are not quite
o wide. For example, we might want to compare pink noise
ith blue noise, or pink noise with white noise. Gerber and
ilner (1971) showed the transitivity of loudness level for
everal one-third octave and one octave bands. It would be

useful for us to examine the equal loudness properties of
these several bands throughout infancy as a measure of development of psychoacoustic function. For example, Bull et al.
(1981) have examined the masking of octave band noise by
broad spectrum noise and found that the thresholds in infants
were 16 to 25 dB greater than the thresholds obtained for
adults. Is this a sensory, perceptual, or cognitive
phenomenon? If we continue to employ bandwidth as our criterion for stimulus complexity, then a world of experiments
on that simple criterion awaits us.

REFERENCES

Bench, J. "Audio-frequency and audio-intensity discrimination in the human neonate" International Audiology
8(4):615-625,1969.

Bench, J., Collyer, Y., Mentz, L. and Wilson, I. "Studies
in infant behavioral audiometry" Audiology 15:85-105,
1976.

Bench, J. and Mentz, L. "Stimulus complexity, state and
infants' auditory behavioral responses" British Journal
of Disorders of Communication 10:52-60, 1975.

Broadbent, D.E. Perception and Communication (Oxford:
Pergamon Press), 1958.

Bull, D., Schneider, B.A. and Trehub, S.E. "The masking of
octave-band noise by broad-spectrum noise in infants"
Perception and Psychophysics 30:101-106, 1981.

Eisenberg, R.B. "Auditory behavior in the human neonate:
functional properties of sound and their ontogenetic
implications" International Audiology 8:34-45, 1969.

Franklin, B. "Audiometric testing using narrow speech bands"
Paper presented at the International Congress on Education of the Deaf, Hamburg, 1980.

Franklin, B. "Newborn responses to acoustic stimuli" Paper
presented at the 102nd meeting of the Acoustical Society
of America, Miami Beach, 1981.

Gerber, S.E. "Neonatal auditory testing: A review" in
Cunningham, G.C. (ed.) Conference on Newborn Hearing
Screening (Berkeley: California State Department of
Public Health), 1971.

Gerber, S.E., Jones, B.L. and Costello, J.M. "Behavioral
measures" in Gerber, S.E. (ed.) Audiometry in Infancy
(New York: Grune & Stratton, Inc.), 1977.

Gerber, S.E., Lima, C.G., and Copriviza, K.L. "Auditory
arousal in preterm infants" Scandinavian Audiology,
in press.

Gerber, S.E. and Mencher, G.T. "Arousal responses of neonates to wide band and narrow band noise" Paper presented
at the Annual Convention of the American Speech-Language-
Hearing Association, Atlanta, 1979.

Gerber, S.E. and Milner, P. "The transitivity of loudness
level" Journal of the Audio Engineering Society 19:
656-659, 1971.

Gerber, S.E., Mulac, A. and Swain, B.J. "Idiosyncratic
cardiovascular response of human neonates to acoustic
stimuli" The Journal of the American Audiology Society
1(5):185-191, 1976.

Hardy, J.D., Hardy, W.G., and Hardy, M.P. "Some problems
in neonatal screening" Trans. Amer. Acad. Ophthalmol.
Otolaryngol 74:1229-1235, 1970.

Johansson, B., Wedenberg, E., and Westin, B. "Measurement
of tone response by the human foetus" Acta Oto-laryngologica 57:188-192, 1964.

Ling, D., Ling, A.H. and Doehring, D.G. "Stimulus, response
and observer variables in the auditory screening of
newborn infants" The Journal of Speech and Hearing
Research 13(1):9-18, 1970.

Mason, LA. "Neonates' responses to loudness-balanced
wide and narrow band acoustic stimuli" Unpublished
Master's thesis, University of California, Santa
Barbara, 1981.

Mencher, G.T. (ed.) Early Identification of Hearing Loss
(Basel: S. Karger), 1976.

Mencher, G.T., Derbyshire, A.V., McCulloch, B. and Dethlefs, R. "Observer bias as a factor in neonatal hearing screening" Paper presented at the Annual Convention of the American Speech and Hearing Association, Detroit, 1973.

Mendel, M.I. "Infant responses to recorded sounds" Journal of Speech and Hearing Research 11:811-816, 1968.

Tanaka, Y. and Arayama, T. "Fetal responses to acoustic stimuli" Practica Oto-Rhinolaryngologica 31:269-273, 1969.

Taylor, D.J. and Mencher, G.T. "Neonate response: the effect of infant state and auditory stimuli" Archives of Otolaryngology 95:120-124, 1972.

AUDITORY BEHAVIOR IN INFANCY

Wesley R. Wilson
University of Washington, Seattle, Washington
and
Sanford E. Gerber
University of California, Santa Barbara

Sound presented to an infant does result in a response; from there on it's pure speculation. Since the title of this volume is development, we first build a case that there is no development in the behavioral responses to audition, and then we talk about what we think is occurring developmentally. In the field of clinical audiology a number of people believe that there's a rather substantial change across age in response to sound. When they talk about development, they talk about changes in clinical baselines that are of really large magnitude. We think it's time to give some evidence that will put to rest some of those contentions.

Figure 7-1 is from Northern and Downs (1978) and is often attributed to Murphy (1961) in terms of the data for it. There really is no data-based paper for it. The paper is one in which he says that he believes that babies do these things. The idea expressed in this figure is that infants first will turn in a horizontal plane, that they'll turn to the right (there will be a bias or loading to the right), and that localization appears at about 4-6 months. Northern and Downs add some localizations in the vertical plane, and they trace this out to about 24 months. So there's a suggestion, then, that localization "develops" at about 4-6 months, that's when it seems to come in strongly, and then the vertical domain is added to the horizontal domain.

A second area is related to the types of measurements that Gerber described in the previous chapter. We would categorize them as a behavioral observation approach; that, as you provide the sound stimulus, you observe overt responses to the stimuli and infer from that some kinds of "threshold" or at least some baseline for clinical purposes. We don't know if you have to deal with the issue of threshold, but very clearly there's a concept that there is some essence of normal. One can learn several things from data over the ages from four months to 24 months. For example, noisemakers

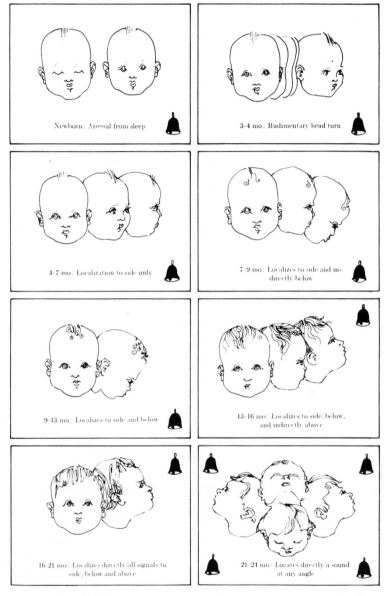

Figure 7-1. Maturation of the auditory response (from Northern and Downs, 1978).

150

are suggesting that, at 4-7 months, babies will respond at
around 50 dB sound pressure level. At 24 months it will be
about 25 dB sound pressure level. So there appears to be a
25 dB shift in response level. For response levels to pure
tones, the change is perhaps even slightly greater and that
led to Gerber's suggestion that pure tones are reasonably
inefficient for this type of testing. For speech the changes
are somewhat slighter, and this led to inferences that speech
was a better signal (Fig. 7-2). There is a suggestion that
there is a developmental change in responses as one goes
through the first 2 years of life. Figure 7-3 (Sweitzer,
1977) shows minimum response levels for speech, and it's
again related to the notion that during the first two years
of life there is a rather dramatic change in the level at
which infants will respond to speech. The hard data come
more from assertions that behavioral responses that are not
reinforced represent some estimate of threshold. In other
words, take a paradigm similar to the one Gerber described
for neonates and apply that across the first two years of
life. Typically what one finds is a very rapid habituation,
so median data are usually taken from a group of infants.
These medians may say that a group of three-month-old infants
respond to the first time a signal is presented at about
60 dB, and the next time around 80 dB, and therefore threshold is 70 dB. They are always group data, there are always
several presentations, and the data are characterized by
extremely wide variance.

Data from the behavioral observation type of approach
(Eisenberg, 1976) suggest that infants' hearing for a 4000
Hz pure tone is poorer than for a 500 Hz tone. This observation suggests that infants' hearing may be poorer in the
high frequencies and better in the low frequencies, but
again these are all unreinforced approaches. In his chapter,
Gerber summarized that literature when he talked about state,
changes in signal, bandwidth, their effects, etc. The result
in clinical approaches that really do not have a baseline
with good enough specificity to allow one to make particular
judgments. That literature also suggested that head turning
behavior develops at about 4-6 months of age, and that certain signals were much more efficient than other signals.

Some recent studies by Muir and his colleagues (1979)
relate to these questions, and persons might wish to look
at his work as a strategy relative to the testing of neonates. Basically what Muir's group did was to look at what
they called head turn behavior, which they later called

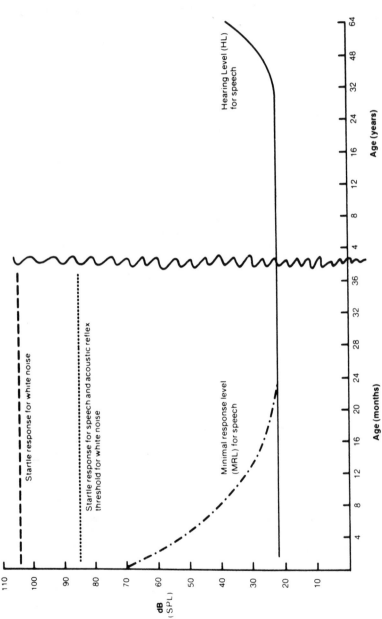

Figure 7-2. Relationships between age in months (to the left of the dividing line) and age in years (to the right of the dividing line) and intensities (dB SPL) necessary to obtain: 1) minimal response level (MRL) for speech, 2) hearing level (HL) for speech, 3) startle response for speech and acoustic reflex threshold for white noise, and 4) startle response for white noise

152

Summary of behavioral test procedures, expected response, and information obtained as a function of age

Age range	Test procedures	Expected response	Information obtained
0 to 4 months	Sound field BOA using noise, voice, music, and environmental sounds	Reflexive behavior: startle response auropalpebral Cessation of activity Initiation of activity	Extent of hearing impairment
5 to 18 months	Sound field BOA, COR, and VRA using same signals as before plus narrow band noise or frequency-modulated pure tones	Same behavioral response as before; look for development of localization to mature by age 1 year	Extent of hearing impairment Frequency characteristics (?) Difference in hearing acuity between ears
15 to 30 months	Same as before; may also attempt identification of body parts; simple pictures; try AC and BC SHL; also try TROCA	Same behavioral response as before; look for development of response of specific verbal commands	Same as before; in addition, may be able to identify type of loss
30 months to 5 years	Same as before; use AC and BC pure tones, SHL, SDL; speech discrimination; may test for auditory perceptual problems	Conditioned response to pure tones; obtaining specific responses to verbal material	Same as before; in addition, can begin to look for auditory perceptual problems

Figure 7-3. Summary of behavioral test procedures, expected response, and information obtained as a function of age (from Sweitzer, 1977).

153

localization behavior because subsequent studies showed a
localization type response. They took two rattles - one had
something to make a sound and the other didn't - and they
activated them to the side of an infant's head and videotaped
the infant. They stretched the response window up to about
15 seconds of behavior, and found that, at birth, a very high
percentage of the infants will turn toward the sound source.
At one month of age even a higher percentage will turn to it;
at two months it drops to chance behavior; at three months
it seems to be coming back. They charted the same babies
over a period of time; three of the four babies showed a very
high response rate at birth. There seems to be a rather rapid
change in terms of head turning behavior.

 A very simple interpretation of these data would have to
be that inferences about localization that suggest it develops
strongly at four-six months may be looking at the recurrence
of head turning behavior as reported by Muir et al. (1979).
This raises several interesting questions. Why does a baby
have a certain type of response behavior drop out over time
and come back in? A cognitive (i.e., maturational) explanation of it (rather than a learning or developmental explanation) follows the line of saying that an infant at birth or
close to birth is responding reflexively, can then move into
sensory-motor type of behavior, and can then move into a
phase using this response to explore the environment. That
intuitively makes more sense than some other explanation.

Inferences about localization and our knowledge about
head turning behavior have to be changed to suggest that
this does show a developmental sequence and that it's present
much earlier than many persons believed it to be. We want to
look at it in terms of what happens if you reinforce the head
turn response. When we talk about head turn behaviors, we
were talking about putting the infant in a sound controlled
environment. We're using earphones, but one can use loud
speakers. We use a visual reinforcer which right now is
animated toys that light up; we simply have a column of them
stacked. This has proven to be a fairly potent paradigm in
terms of increasing infant behavior. The first study is the
one that Moore did which examined the effect of reinforcement
on this head turn behavior (Moore and Wilson, 1978). In all
of the studies that we do that make use of this paradigm,
we include signal presentations and control trials. The
purpose of the control trial is to exclude data from any
infant who goes beyond a false response rate which suggests
that the data may be questionable. The judgments are very

simple. The infant makes a turn or does not. They use two
judges; inter-judge agreement is always about 95%. The signal in this study was a 70 dB shaped noise with the predomi-
nant energy from 500 to 2000 Hz; it's a masking signal that's
used rather routinely on a number of audiometers. We use it
simply because the works that Gerber talked about in the
previous chapter suggested that a masking noise was a reasonably decent signal when you're eliciting responses. What
we played with was response behavior. Referring to Fig. 7-4,
one notices that with reinforcement, there are about 4-5
responses from the infant. If one continues presentations at
a fixed level, in this case 70 dB sound pressure level, there
is a gain of another 5 responses out of the remaining 25
presentations. Social reinforcement increases the response
rate slightly. With simple visual reinforcement, in this
case a flashing light, there is an increased response rate.
Finally, with a complex reinforcer, which was the toy, the
data get very close to a one-to-one response rate for
stimulus presentation. The mean is on the order of 27 of
30 for 12-18 month olds. We continue the same type of study
looking at younger ages. Here we used only two conditions:
complex visual reinforcer and no reinforcement. At around
four months of age having reinforcement substantially increases the response behavior. These data are in direct
contrast to Muir's (1979) data because at four months he was
finding 100% response rate with no reinforcement. Remember
he's using a paradigm where he allows an unlimited window,
which Trehub and Schneider discuss in Chapter 8. He uses a
turn right-turn left response. We think that's a distinct
advantage of Trehub's and Muir's approach to it: allow the
babies long enough to respond and they will show you meaningful behavior. Using visual reinforcement will give
response behavior that is dramatically different from not
using reinforcement with infants from 4½ months of age on
up. The simple act of adding visual reinforcement permits
us to get responses to a signal that approach a 100% response
rate; i.e., on the order of 25-30 responses to 25-30
presentations.

Another way of looking at the same sort of thing is in
a single subject design where you introduce reinforcement,
remove reinforcement, reintroduce it, etc. In Fig. 7-5 are
two subjects at six months of age; they're reinforced,
they're responding at a 100% rate. Reinforcement is removed
after the 5th trial; and then they diminish and quit responding. They simply show no responses to the sound, 70 dB
sound pressure level, broad band noise. They give a negative

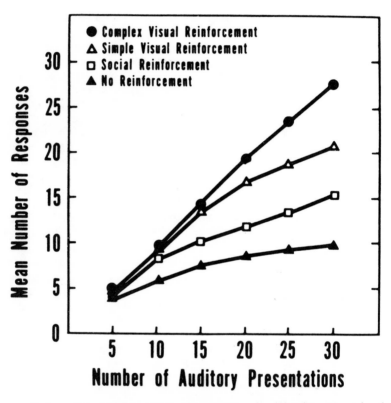

Figure 7-4. Cumulative mean responses in blocks of stimulus trials for four reinforcement conditions with N=12 in each group (from Moore, Thompson, and Thompson, 1975).

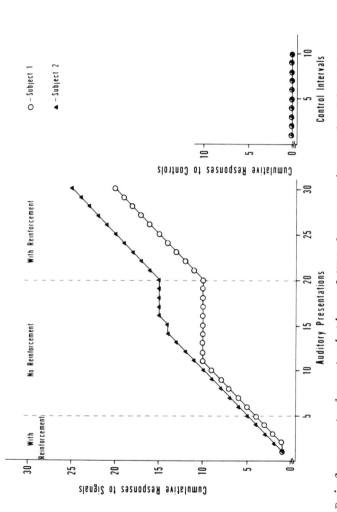

Figure 7-5. Reinforcement characteristics of VRA for two six-month-old subjects on single subject reversal design. Reinforcement provided for correct response (head turn) on presentations 1-5; removed presentations 6-20; 21 used as teaching trial with paired stimulus and reinforcement; and reinforcement available again on 22-30 (from Moore and Wilson, 1978).

157

response, they try one more positive, they do get paid off,
they give negative responses. Following the 20th presentation, they gave one teaching trial - which simply says the
signal goes on, a second later the reinforcer comes on - and
both infants then gave 10 out of 10 responses with reinforcement. So it's the single subject design that is more acceptable in terms of demonstration of strength of reinforcement,
but it gives the same evidence as the earlier ones.

How do we relate these data to thresholds? First of all,
in Figure 7-6 are "threshold estimations" using an approach
without reinforcement-behavioral observation approach. The
critical information is that the range is from the tenth to
the ninetieth percentile. These are data developed by
Thompson and Weber (1974). Their interpretation is identical
to ours, and that is that the behavioral observation approach
cannot be used in any way to describe threshold. Take the
clinical difficulty here. Do you interpret that babies have
normal hearing because they're in the range of the tenth to
the ninetieth percentile? Using the head turn procedures
we've described, looking across stages, again to a complex
noise, we find that the range of our 10th to 90th percentiles
is reduced to one measurement step (Fig. 7-7). The measurement steps in this case were 10 dB; so the 10th to 90th
percentile is at either 20 dB or 30 dB across ages. Clinically, then, we would say that if one sees infants with
this procedure in a test room with a loud speaker and this
signal - because signal parameters are dramatic in sound
field testing - that if they do not respond at 30 dB levels
they should be followed.

We said earlier we'd come back to some concept of development. There is no development for clinical purposes. You
don't have an idea that, when you see a six-month-old, you
add a 30 dB correction factor because of the dramatic change
in hearing over the first years of life. Is this a developmental trend? The next study used pure tones and its purpose
was to compare earphone and sound field testing. There are
two things we think are important about it. First of all,
pure tones have some utility in assessment of hearing sensitivity and previous work has suggested pure tones can't be
used. The utility is obvious and gives information that is
frequency specific. The second thing was that we wanted to
test under earphones because there is a number of auditory
questions that can't be posed properly in a sound field
environment. Even threshold in a sound field environment
is very problematic particularly at high frequencies, and

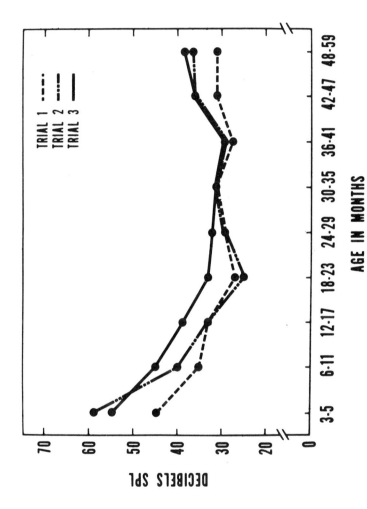

Figure 7-6. Median response curves in decibels sound pressure level for three test trials as a function of age (from Thompson and Weber, 1974).

159

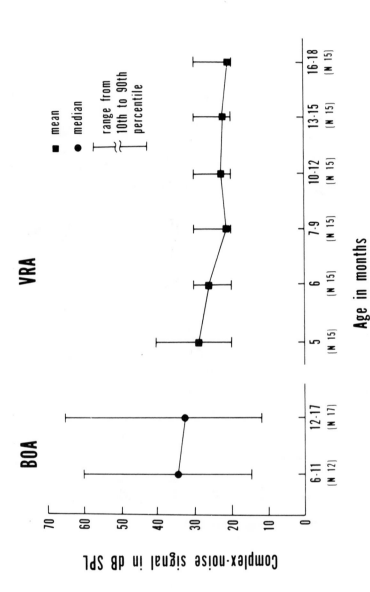

Figure 7-7. Soundfield auditory thresholds of infants as obtained by BOA and VRA methods as a function of age (from Moore and Wilson, 1978).

so we are interested in solving two things: one, coupling an
earphone in such a way that one can get a behavioral response
that is meaningful; and, two, using pure tone signals. We
used the warble pure tone because in a sound field presentation there is less variation as a function of location in
space. We used three groups, six to seven month old infants,
12-13 month old infants, and an adult group and selected
3 frequencies, 500, 1000, and 4000 Hz. Table 7-1 shows the
infant data; the ranges are the full range, not the 10th to
90th percentile. Again the measurement step size here is
10 dB. We did not see a significant difference between the
six-month-old and the 12-month-old, but again the measurement
step might mask that. The process required of infants is
identical to the process required of adults, it's a minimum
of 3 correct responses out of 6. The first thing we can
infer from this, then, is that 4000 Hz is not inherently a
signal that infants do not respond to. It is the signal
that infants prefer not to respond to. Hoversten and Moncur
(1969) said that infants are much more responsive at 500 Hz
than at 4000 Hz; that simply isn't true when you change the
paradigm. We don't mean that their data are wrong; we are
saying that paradigms are specific.

Young adults show wider dispersion than infants: the
infant dispersion data are equal to or better than young
adults. We don't have to make allowances for infants in
terms of the dispersion of data. Younger infants show poorer
hearing than older infants at 500 Hz. The sound field data
didn't show it and the earphone data did show it. Earphone
coupling probably plays a significant role here. At both
1000 Hz and 4000 Hz we see the six-month-old infants start to
separate out; whereas, in the sound field, at one frequency
the younger ones had better thresholds, in another, the older
ones did.

Frequency separation becomes greater between adults
and infants, which raises the whole question of whether
infants' hearing may be better at the high frequencies and
poorer in the low frequencies as evidenced by behavioral
procedures. Why use the adult as a model in terms of what
development should be charted against? It could simply be
that adults are losing high frequency hearing. We spend a
lot of time looking at infants, and have developed an argument that low frequency hearing is poor in 6-month-old
infants but appears to be approaching adult norms at 12
months of age. Elliott and Katz (1980) showed a developmental trend between 6 years and 10 years of age with 10-year-

TABLE 7-1. *Range of responses from the 10th to 90th percentile and mean response levels for 19 infants between six and 13 months of age (from Moore and Wilson, 1978).*

		EARPHONE			SOUNDFIELD		
		500 Hz	1000 Hz	4000 Hz	500 Hz	1000 Hz	4000 Hz
6-7 MONTH OLD	MEAN IN dB SPL	37.5	25.0	22.5	17.5	17.5	16.3
	RANGE IN dB	30-40	20-30	20-30	10-20	10-20	10-20
12-13 MONTH OLD	MEAN IN dB SPL	31.4	27.1	25.0	21.1	15.6	14.4
	RANGE IN dB	30-40	20-30	20-30	20-30	10-20	10-20

olds having reached adult values. Yoneshige and Elliott
(1981) reported on 6-year-olds and adults. The only difference reported from Elliott and Katz is that Yoneshige and
Elliott screened tympanometrically and excluded persons with
abnormal tympanometry. There's a dramatic shift, 10 dB,
between six-year-olds tested by the same procedure in the
same laboratory and adults tested at the same procedure in
the same laboratory.

Nozza (1981) did an adaptive procedure of 5 dB step size
with infants that was very similar to what Elliott and colleagues have done. Since he did tympanometric screening
after he had collected all of the other data, he had the data
for babies who passed an oral screen, a history, but failed
a tympanometry screen. He used a very stringent tympanometry
criterion, ± 50 millimeters. If the tympanometric peak moved
outside of ± 50 millimeters, they were excluded. Obviously,
if they had no peak they were excluded. The shift in threshold between the group which includes those who passed an
oral screen but failed the tympanometric screening and those
who passed both screens is 5 dB at 1000 or 4000 Hz. In an
adaptive test procedure it shifts thresholds 5 dB by that
simple thing. If you come back, then, to Elliott's data,
maybe the difference between the two studies is at least partially assignable to the exclusion of individuals with changes
in middle ear pressure. The shift in the thresholds reported in earlier studies might differ on the order of 5 dB
because of a failure to screen tympanometrically and compare that to adult data, it brings our infants to within
about 3-4 dB of adults, but it does vary somewhat as a function of frequency. That is clearly an area of further
research where those data have to be included and dealt
with in terms of other clinical implications. We're saying
now something as simple as a tympanometric screen will dramatically shift threshold estimations for infants.

As we look at the data that we tried to present, and as we
look at the data that other persons are presenting in this
volume, we think that our argument should focus more on questions related to strategies adopted or cognitive styles
adopted, and the developmental changes in audition should be
studied more from the point of view of cognitive changes and
less from the point of view of sensory changes. We believe,
however, that it would be quite easy to answer the sensory
change questions now. We think the methodology has reached
the point where that can be done; the study can be done to
look at developmental changes by following a group of children

as they themselves develop instead of a cross section. We
think we can make reasonable inferences about the sensory
changes, and we think that work is going on in several laboratories and will be available in the next few years. The more
interesting work will rest with things that suggest whether
changes between six and 12-month-olds are in terms of the
strategies they adopt in resolving this particular auditory
task. We think the answer is definitely yes, there is. Again
Nozza's dissertation shows that 12-month-olds are much more
efficient in arriving at criterion. We can demonstrate
changes. We used a fixed trial response task. When a change
occurs, be it a speech stimulus or a pure tone stimulus, the
infants will show an immediate response to it that is scor-
able reliably, and they'll wait until the end of the response
interval to turn their head and receive the payoff. They've
simply mastered and learned the fact that they are going to
get three tokens, and they can wait until the third one if
they want to because they're more interested in what the
assistant is doing and they're going to get paid off. They
can win at the game. And it's very clear that the infants
are using auditory information to modify cognitive strategies
and they're playing with it in ways none of our procedures
is addressing at all right now, but they can be addressed.
We hope that we can also tie together some of the electro-
physiologic data with the behavioral data, but we are much
less optimistic about that than two or three years
ago. We followed Down's Syndrome infants and normally developing infants for three years, both electrophysiologically
and behaviorally, and we simply don't see any sort of
organizational framework (Wilson et al., in press). So we
believe that we have to look at the effect of methodology
on the results, we have to translate the results as a function of the methodologies, we believe that behaviorally we've
moved a reasonably good distance in resolving some of the
methodological issues. We think there are several methodological studies that remain to be done, and they're fairly
straightforward. We think we can then get on to charting
the sensory changes which we haven't discussed, but one can
go beyond anything related to sensitivity. We've done
studies on the critical ratio, masking studies. We've done
studies on simple processing. We think there's a fair amount
of excitement that answers can be derived behaviorally that
will show a sort of robustness and stand up to comparison,
and much can be learned about the auditory system.

REFERENCES

Eisenberg, R.B. Auditory Competence in Early Life. Baltimore:
University Park Press, 1976.

Elliott, L.L. and Katz, D.R. "Children's Pure-Tone Detection"
J. Acoust. Soc. Amer. 67: 343-344, 1980.

Gerber, S.E. "Auditory behavior in the neonatal period,"
this volume.

Hoversten, G.H. and Moncur, J.P. "Stimuli and intensity
factors in testing infants," Journal of Speech and
Hearing Research, 12, 687-702, 1969.

Moore, J.M., Thompson, G. and Thompson, M. "Auditory
localization of infants as a function of reinforcement
conditions," Journal of Speech and Hearing Disorders,
40, 29-34, 1975.

Moore, J.M. and Wilson, W.R. "Visual reinforcement audio-
metry (VRA) with infants," in S.E. Gerber and G.T.
Mencher (eds.), Early Diagnosis of Hearing Loss. New
York: Grune and Stratton, Inc., 1978.

Muir, D., Abraham, W., Forbes, B., and Harris, L. "The
ontogenesis of an auditory localization response from
birth to four months of age" Canadian Journal of
Psychology 33, 320-333, 1979.

Muir, D. and Field, J. "Newborn infants orient to sounds,"
Child Development 50, 431-436, 1979.

Murphy, K.P. "Development of hearing in babies," Hearing
News 29, 9-11, 1961.

Northern, J.L. and Downs, M.P. Hearing in Children (2nd
ed.). Baltimore: Williams and Wilkins, 1978.

Nozza, R.J. "Detection of pure tones in quiet and in noise
by infants and adults," unpublished doctoral dissertation, University of Washington, 1981.

Sweitzer, R.S. "Audiologic evaluation of the infant and
young child" in B.F. Jaffe (ed.) Hearing Loss in
Children. Baltimore: University Park Press, 1977.

Thompson, G. and Weber, B.A.   "Responses of infants and
    young children to behavior observation audiometry,"
    Journal of Speech and Hearing Disorders 39, 140-147,
    1974.

Trehub, S.E. and Schneider, B.A.   "Recent advances in the
    behavioral study of infant audition," this volume

Wilson, W.R., Folsom, R.C. and Widen, J.E.   "Hearing impair-
    ment in Down syndrome children," in G.T. Mencher and
    S.E. Gerber (eds.), The Multiply-Handicapped Hearing
    Impaired Child. New York: Grune and Stratton, Inc.,
    in press.

Yoneshige, Y. and Elliott, L.L.   "Pure-tone sensitivity and
    ear canal pressure at threshold in Children and Adults"
    J. Acoust. Soc. Amer. 70: 1272-1276, 1981.

Recent Advances in the Behavioral Study of Infant Audition

Sandra E. Trehub and Bruce A. Schneider
University of Toronto, Mississauga, Ontario

The recent surge of research interest in infant audition
has generated new empirical and methodological insights (see
Schneider, Trehub, and Bull, 1979; Trehub, Bull, and Schneider,
1981b for reviews). Nevertheless, our knowledge of developmental changes in basic auditory processes remains primitive.
Studies of infants and young children have generally been
limited in scope, focusing on a narrow range of ages and signals. Where age comparisons have been potentially feasible,
either within or across studies, these have been impeded by
the typical use of divergent methods across age groups.

In our own laboratory, we (Bruce Schneider, Dale Bull,
and I) have been attempting to make some headway in mapping
the developmental course of basic auditory abilities from six
months onwards. To this end, we have tested thousands of
infants over the past few years. In this chapter I outline
some of our findings to date as well as some of our future
directions. Finally, I offer comments on potential applications of this work.

The cornerstone of our data-gathering efforts is our
procedure, which is a refinement of the visual reinforcement
audiometry procedures used in numerous research and clinical
settings. The basis of this technique is a localization
response or orientation of head and eyes toward a sound
source. In contrast to Wilson and others (e.g., Moore,
Thompson, and Thompson, 1975; Wilson, 1978; Wilson, this
volume) who have used a left-turning response toward a single
loudspeaker, we use two possible responses (left or right
turning) and two loudspeakers. Moreover, in preference to
the fixed response interval in general use, we have substi-
tuted an unlimited response interval coupled with forced-
choice responding. What we have, then, is a two-alternative,
forced-choice, signal-detection task that eliminates the need
for control (no-stimulus) trials, minimizes concerns about

167

response bias, and accommodates infants who may be slow to
respond.

During an experimental session, both the mother, seated
on the test chair, and the infant, placed on her lap, face
an experimenter seated in the opposite corner of a sound-
attenuating booth. Loudspeakers are located 45 degrees off
midline to the infant's right and left. Both the mother and
the experimenter wear headphones over which masking noise is
presented to prevent them from detecting the locus of a test
signal. A trial is initiated only when the infant is quiet
and looking directly ahead. A signal (e.g., a narrow-band
noise) is then presented at one of the two speakers and it
remains on until the infant makes a head turn of 45 degrees
or more toward either side. If the head turn is in the direction of the speaker producing the signal, the signal is turned
off and a toy (or T.V.) above (or beside) that speaker is
illuminated and activated for a period of four seconds. If
the head turn is in a direction away from that speaker, the
signal is also turned off and there is a 4-second silent
interval. In all cases, the signal remains on until a head
turn occurs. To ensure that all of the infants can perform
the task of turning to the sound location, a training criterion
is employed with sound intensity well above threshold. During
the training period, the location of the signal is alternated
between left and right speakers until the child makes four
successive, correct responses. The intensity is then reduced
5 or 10 dB and the alternation continues until the infant
again makes four successive, correct responses. When this
training criterion is reached, the actual test series begins.
Typically, more than 95% of infants from 6 to 24 months of
age satisfy this criterion readily, and usually 85-90% complete a session on a single visit without fussing or crying.
During a typical test session, five different intensity levels
of the signal are presented a total of five times each. The
five intensity levels and the two sound locations are random-
ized over trials. At the conclusion of the first session,
we often attempt a second session in order to maximize the
amount of information obtained from any infant. At the
beginning of the second session, training is repeated as
before with the exception that only two successive, correct
responses are required at each intensity level.

In our continuing efforts to interest even more infants
for ever longer periods of time, we devote much energy to
potential improvements in the entertainment (i.e., reinforcement) aspect of our procedure. Our most recent reinforcer

comprises, in part, a dark glass enclosure with four different toys that can be illuminated and activated independently in random order (Figs. 8-1a and 8-1b). If boredom sets in, we change over to color television monitors that are adjacent to each of the boxes. The televisions, when operative, deliver 4-second pre-recorded segments of lively audio-visual output from Sesame Street and the like.

Formal testing has largely been restricted to infants 6 to 24 months of age and adults, but pilot testing with other ages has convinced us of the applicability of our procedure throughout the life span. Moreover, our data from adult subjects are comparable to those obtained with more typical psychophysical procedures (Bull, Schneider, and Trehub, 1981).

Formal Evaluation of our Procedure

As noted, the various studies of auditory acuity in infancy have been characterized by methodological diversity. Neonates have been the typical population of interest (e.g., Crowell et al., 1971; Engel and Young, 1969; Hutt et al., 1968) but not the only target population (e.g., Bench et al., 1976; Schulman and Wade, 1970; Schneider, Trehub, and Bull, 1980; Trehub, Schneider, and Endman, 1980). Physiological or autonomic responses have been used most frequently (e.g., Crowell et al., 1971; Hutt et al., 1968) but not exclusively (e.g., Thompson and Weber, 1974; Trehub et al., 1980), and the responses, physiological or behavioral, have mostly been unreinforced. Finally, the stimuli in most studies of infant audition have been brief (5 seconds or less) and the response interval has generally been of fixed duration. This contrasts with the unlimited stimulus and response intervals character-istic of our procedure.

We investigated the implications of two of these pro-cedural variables, reinforcement and response interval, on the assessment of infants' auditory sensitivity (Trehub, Schneider, and Bull, 1981). First, we modified our standard procedure by eliminating reinforcement and introducing a 5-second response interval. Immediately following a test session with these changes, we retested the infants with our standard procedure, with reinforcement and the unlimited response interval reinstated. The stimuli were octave-band noises with center frequencies of 400 or 4,000 Hz. The per-centage of correct head turns as a function of the decibel

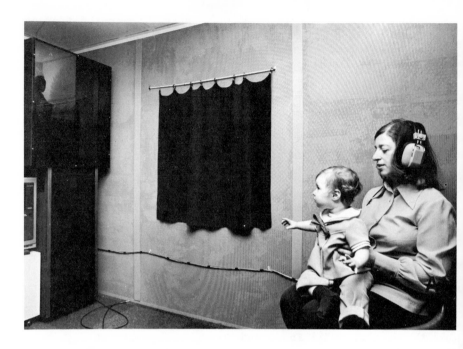

Figure 8-1a. Partial view of sound booth

level of the two test frequencies is shown in Figure 8-2. Each
data point is based on 100 trials. For the reinforced conditions, at least, correct responses increase as the intensity
of the signal increases. The psychometric functions for the
nonreinforced conditions are dramatically lower than those
of the reinforced conditions for the 400 and 4000 Hz stimuli.
In a subsequent experiment, we sought to separate the influence of reinforcement from that of response interval. The
first test session again involved nonreinforcement and a 5-
second response interval. In the second session, the same
response interval prevailed but reinforcement was added. As
can be seen in Fig. 8-3 (where each data point is based on
160 trials for the 400 Hz stimulus and 180 trials for the
4000 Hz stimulus), the omission of reinforcement impairs performance for both stimuli, but the impairment is not as dramatic as in the previous experiment. The specific effect of
the limited response interval can be seen more clearly in
Fig. 8-4 where the psychometric functions from the reinforcement conditions of both experiments are shown. Changing from
an unlimited response interval to one of 5 seconds impairs

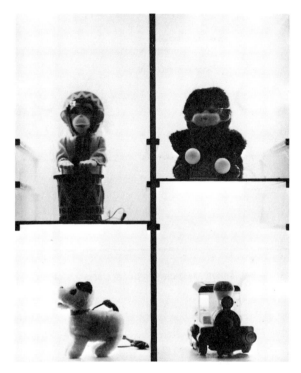

Figure 8-1b. The reinforcers

performance at both frequencies. The beneficial effects of the unlimited response interval indicate that the majority of long-latency responses are, nevertheless, correct responses. The nonreinforced session not only resulted in fewer correct responses than the reinforced session but also produced substantially fewer head turns overall.

Thus we have clear evidence of sounds that are perceptible, as shown in the prior reinforced session, but that nevertheless fail to yield correct responses, as shown in the nonreinforced session with the same infants. Without reinforcement, many of the lower intensity stimuli fail to capture the attention of the infant. By reinforcing responses to our test stimuli, however, we confer these stimuli with significance of attention-eliciting properties. In so doing, we maximize our chances of approximating the "true" detection threshold. It would therefore appear that the omission of reinforcement or the inclusion of a fixed response interval

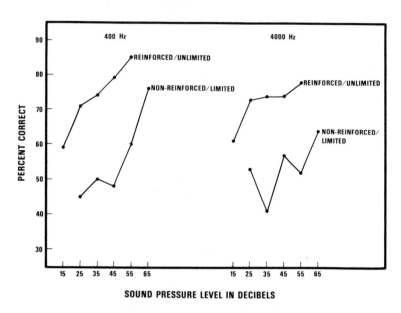

Figure 8-2.   Percentage of correct head turns as a function of decibel level of two test frequencies and of reinforcement or nonreinforcement. From Trehub, Schneider, and Bull (1981).

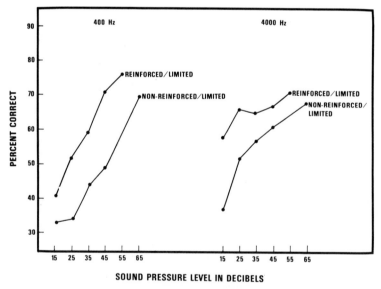

Figure 8-3.   Percentage of correct head turns as a function of decibel level of two test frequencies and of reinforcement or nonreinforcement.   From Trehub, Schneider, and Bull (1981).

172

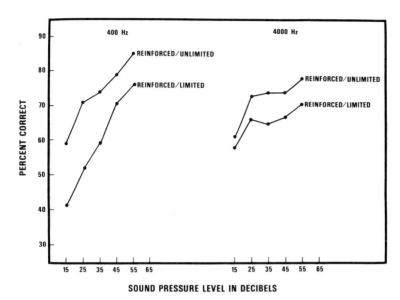

Figure 8-4. Percentage of correct head turns as a function of decibel level of two test frequencies and of unlimited or limited response intervals for reinforcement conditions of both experiments. From Trehub, Schneider, and Bull (1981).

results in substantial underestimation of infants' hearing proficiency.

Absolute Thresholds

For group data gathered with our procedure, we define threshold as the intensity at which the signal is detected 65% of the time. We have demonstrated elsewhere (Trehub et al., 1980) that the 65% correct level is significantly better than chance responding (50%) and is, therefore, clearly audible. Moreover, we have shown that inattentiveness has a greater effect on estimates of stimulus detectability at higher than at lower intensities.

We have provided extensive normative data on infants'
thresholds for narrow band noises with center frequencies
ranging from 200 Hz to 19,000 Hz (Schneider et al., 1980;
Trehub et al., 1980). In short, we found that infant-adult
differences were greatest at the lower frequencies (approximately 20-25 dB) and decreased at higher frequencies, dis-
appearing finally at 19,000 Hz. This convergence at very
high frequencies can be seen in the psychometric functions of
Fig. 8-5 and corresponding thresholds of Fig. 8-6. These
findings indicate that developmental changes beyond six months
of age must comprise considerable improvement in stimulus
detection at the lower frequencies.

Thresholds in Noise Backgrounds: Masking

We adapted our procedure to permit the determination of
thresholds for specific signals in a background of broad band
noise. The procedure remained as before except that a

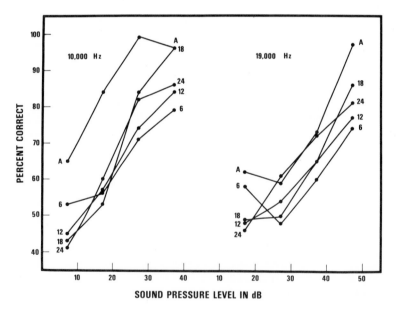

*Figure 8-5. Percentage of correct head turns as a function of
decibel level of half-octave band noises with center frequencies of 10,000 and 19,000 Hz for infants 6, 12, 18, and 24
months of age and for adults. From Schneider, Trehub, and
Bull (1980).*

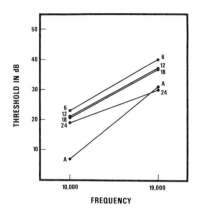

Figure 8-6. Thresholds for half-octave band noises with center frequencies of 10,000 and 19,000 Hz for infants 6, 12, 18, and 24 months of age and four adults. From Schneider, Trehub, and Bull (1980).

background noise was present continuously on both loudspeakers. In one study, our signal was a recorded phrase ("Hi there") and infants (6 to 24 months of age) and adults were tested under two levels of masking noise, 42 and 60 dBC (Trehub, Bull, and Schneider, 1981). Thresholds for the speech signal were comparable across all infant groups for both levels of masking noise. Increasing the masking noise from 42 to 60 dBC resulted in a threshold shift of comparable magnitude for infants and adults but infant thresholds were approximately 10-12 dB higher than those of adults at both masking levels (see Fig. 8-7).

In a second experiment with infants 6, 12, 18, and 24 months of age and adults, we studied the detectability of a 4000 Hz octave band noise in the same two noise levels, 42 and 60 dBC (Bull, Schneider, and Trehub, 1981). Masked thresholds were similar for the three older infant groups but were 7-8 dB higher for the 6-month-olds (Fig. 8-8). Again, the effect of increasing the masker by 18 dB was to raise thresholds approximately 18 dB. This is in line with Hawkins and Stevens' (1950) classic finding that an x dB increase in masking noise results in an x dB increase in masked threshold. Thresholds for infants were approximately 20 dB (16-25 dB)

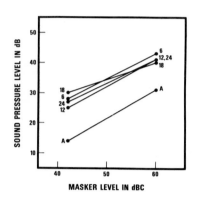

Figure 8-7. Thresholds as a function of masking level for infants 6, 12, 18, and 24 months of age and for adults. From Trehub, Bull, and Schneider (1981a).

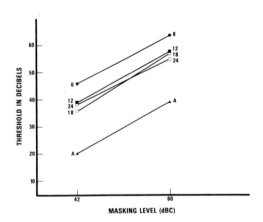

Figure 8-8. Thresholds as a function of masking level for infants 6, 12, 18, and 24 months of age and for adults. From Bull, Schneider, and Trehub (1981).

176

igher than those of adults at both masking levels. This
ompares with a difference of approximately 10 dB in the
peech-masking experiment. Our previous work indicates that
dult-infant differences are smaller for some frequencies than
thers; thus this discrepancy is not problematic. A speech
ignal has its energy spread over a broad frequency range,
nd the detection of such a signal would depend on its most
etectable component. Furthermore, the intensity of a natural
peech signal would be variable in contrast to a band noise.
he calibration of our speech signal was with respect to its
verage intensity.

These masking results, taken together, have implications
or infants' auditory performance in everyday situations. The
ncreased intensity level that infants required for signal
etectability (relative to adults) raises the possibility
hat, in moderately noisy environments, infants may fail to
erceive some signals that are clearly audible for adults.
nfant performance on some listening tasks may be even more
mpaired relative to adults, particularly in situations where
ontext and predictability contribute to signal detectability
Elliott, 1979). Mills (1975) has argued that current levels
f environmental noise are sufficient to interfere with
peech, language, and listening skills in children, but
vidence in support of this claim is limited.

Intensity Difference Thresholds

In order to determine the minimal increase in intensity
hat infants and adults can detect, we adapted our two-
lternative, forced-choice procedure in the following way.
s in the masking experiments, a constant background noise
0-5,000 Hz bandwidth) was presented over both loudspeakers.
he signal in this case, however, was a noise having the same
ower spectrum as the background noise.

In two recently completed experiments (Schneider, Bull,
nd Trehub, in preparation), we studied infants' (12 months)
nd adults' detection of correlated and uncorrelated noise.
n the correlated-noise condition, the added noise was from
he same noise generator as the background noise; in the un-
orrelated condition, the added increment of noise was from
n independent signal generator (The literature suggests that
hresholds for such signals should differ; see Colburn and
urlach, 1978; Durlach and Colburn, 1978). For the indepen-
ent noise source, infants detected a 1.5 dB increment in

noise against a 40 dB background noise and a 0.8 dB increment
in a 60 dB background noise. Infants also detected correlated
noise increments but with less precision. Adults were more
sensitive than infants in both conditions and they showed a
greater difference in their detection of uncorrelated compared to correlated increments.

Individual Thresholds

We have adapted a set of statistical decision procedures
known by the acronym PEST (Parameter Estimation by Sequential
Testing; Taylor and Creelman, 1967) for the determination of
thresholds in individual infants (Bull, Trehub, and Schneider
in preparation). These procedures, used widely in adult
psychophysics, are designed to achieve an accurate threshold
estimate in a relatively brief test session. These modifi-
cations of PEST have been used with our two-alternative,
forced-choice procedure and are geared to the specific problems associated with the testing of infants. Our PEST procedure is fully automated and under micro-computer control.

Basically, PEST searches for the stimulus level that
corresponds to a specified level of detection, say 75%,
which is the level we use. It accumulates evidence on correct
and incorrect responses to guide decisions and increasing or
decreasing the intensity level in order to move closer to
the targeted response probability. The decision history
(continuations and reversals) determines the step size of
subsequent increments or decrements. The final estimate is
achieved when the next change in stimulus level would be
smaller than the minimum step size determined by the experimenter (2 dB for our purposes).

Extensive computer simulations and infant testing indicate that with 20-40 trials an accurate threshold estimate
can be achieved. The simulations indicate that the standard
deviation of 100 estimated thresholds is decreased by less
than 5 dB if the test session is extended to approximately
70 trials.

Our success in collecting individual thresholds can be
illustrated with a study of 18-month-old infants using a
4,000 Hz octave band of noise. These infants were tested on
two different occasions, at least one week apart. When we
consider those infants who completed at least 20 trials in
both sessions, the correlation between the two thresholds
is .82 (see Fig. 8-9).

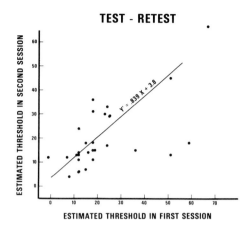

TEST - RETEST

ESTIMATED THRESHOLD IN FIRST SESSION

Figure 8-9.   Test and retest thresholds for a 4,000 Hz octave band of noise by 18-month-old infants.

In Figure 8-10, we can see a graphic representation of a PEST run for N.D., an 18-month-old infant who was tested with a 4,00 Hz octave band of noise. The first four trials represent initial training and N.D. achieves four in a row correct, meeting the intial requirements of training. The signal is then reduced by 10 dB until the criterion of four consecutive, correct responses is met. Again, this happens in four trials. Training is now complete.

The actual test trials begin with the signal being reduced by 8 dB. Initially, we use a relatively lax criterion in order to move to the general vicinity of the infant's threshold. In this phase of testing, the signal intensity is dropped by 8 dB until the infant gets two out of three trials incorrect at a particular level or until the next drop would bring the stimulus intensity to 15 dB. When either of these events takes place, the PEST phase of the session begins. The subsequent trial and every fifth trial are used as a check on attention, at which time the signal is presented at the original training intensity, 65 dB in this case. N.D. is correct on all of these suprathreshold trials.

The PEST phase begins at the level stopped in the previous phase of testing, 15 dB for N.D. Now the infant gets four in a row correct, exceeding 75% correct, so we decrease the intensity by 4 dB, our initial step size in the PEST phase. At 11 dB, N.D. again gets four in a row correct, so

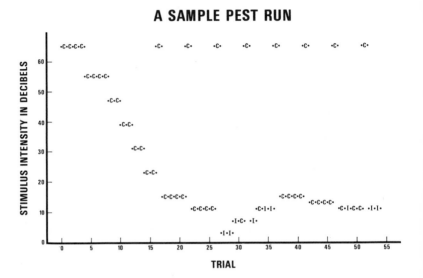

Figure 8-10. Test protocol showing sequence of correct (C) and incorrect (I) responses of an 18-month-old infant.

the intensity must be reduced. Since this is the second intensity change in the same direction, PEST doubles the step
size to 8 dB. (In our selection of PEST parameters, 8 dB is
the maximum step size.) At 3 dB, N.D. gets two incorrect,
necessitating an increase in intensity. Since this is a
reversal, PEST halves the current step size, increasing the
intensity by 4 dB. At 7 dB, N.D. gets two of three trials
incorrect, again less than the targeted probability. Since
there has been a recent reversal, the step size is not doubled
but is increased by the current step size, 4 dB. Again, N.D.
gets 2 out of 3 incorrect, and the stimulus intensity is
increased by 4 dB. At 15 dB, N.D. gets four in a row correct
so the level must be dropped. Since this is a change in
direction, the step size is halved to 2 dB. AT 13 dB, N.D.
gets another four consecutive trials correct, so the intensity
is dropped by the current step size, 2 dB. AT 11 dB, N.D.
gets three incorrect in six trials. This is less than 75%
correct and warrants an increase in intensity. This change
is a reversal, so the step size would be halved to 1 dB. But
we have specified a minimum step size of 2 dB, so PEST simply
terminates the session. The final intensity value that PEST
would have tested, 12 dB, is our estimate of N.D.'s threshold

for the 4,000 Hz band of noise.   Notice that, for all stimulus
levels below 12 dB, N.D.'s performance is no better than 60%
correct, but for all levels above 12 dB, performance is at
100% correct.

Our Future Research Directions

We plan to continue gathering normative and individual
data with our two-alternative, forced-choice technique. Specifically, we intend to map, in detail, the ontogenesis of
basic auditory abilities from six months to six years of age
or until the adult level of skill has been attained.   Thus,
we will pursue studies of absolute thresholds, masked thresholds, intensity-increment thresholds, and individual thresholds over this extended age span.   Furthermore, we are currently enlarging our sample beyond normal infants and children
to include three populations that are at particular risk for
hearing loss: Down's Syndrome and low-birth-weight (less than
1500 grams) infants and children, as well as children who
have been exposed to high levels of environmental noise for
prolonged periods.   Low-birth-weight infants, in addition to
problems associated with general immaturity and poor health,
face further risk through prolonged exposure to incubator
noise (Falk and Farmer, 1973; Peltzman et al., 1970).

In addition to our attempts to clarify empirical and
theoretical questions relevant to this research domain, we
would like to address questions of particular relevance to
the clinic.   To this end, we invite clinicians and clinical
researchers to articulate questions and concerns that we can
address with our collection of research tools.

Practical Applications

We believe that many aspects of the research program
described here have relevance beyond the ivory towers of
academic research.   On the methodological front, we have
demonstrated that reinforcement contributes substantially to
the accuracy of any estimate of hearing proficiency (Trehub,
Schneider, and Bull, 1981).   It is nevertheless the case that
many clinics, including those associated with major university-
affiliated hospitals, do not reinforce the behavioral responses
measured or use ineffective reinforcers.   We have shown, further, that an unlimited response interval can contribute to
the precision of the threshold estimate.   In this regard, some
clinical settings use a fixed response interval; others use an

unspecified, intuitively-determined response interval that
varies from tester to tester and occasion to occasion.

Unfortunately, visits to numerous clinics have revealed
that some rudimentary aspects of standard research practice
are violated routinely. For example, the clinician who
records and interprets responses is typically aware not only
of the occurrence of a trial but also the intensity of the
signal. Moreover, it is relatively rare to find a predetermined protocol for the progression or sequencing of intensity
levels or the number of presentations at each level. Accordingly, judgments of chance responding are intuitive, if they
are made at all. The emergence of control procedures to
circumvent these potential difficulties has been motivated
largely by research demands for "clean" data. Surely the
needs of the clinic are at least as great in this respect.

It is interesting to note that our procedures, by virtue
of their automation, require only a single tester who remains
with the infant and makes very simple judgments about head
orientation--that the infant is facing directly ahead and is
therefore ready for a test trial, or that the infant has made
a 45 degree head turn to the right or left. The sequencing
and alteration of sound levels, the delivery of reinforcers,
and the provision of a permanent record of responses are all
accomplished simply and automatically with the aid of an in-
expensive microcomputer. The programming of the microcomputer
can embody the insights of the most experienced audiologist
or researcher. This eases demands on the tester and yields
a maximally uniform and replicable estimate of hearing status.
In the absence of a microcomputer, a prearranged test protocol
coupled with forced-choice responding provides an acceptable
alternative.

These methodological applications are currently available
for clinical use. In the long run, we hope to make further
contributions to clinical practice by providing norms for
signals relevant to the audiological examination of infants
and young children. This would replace the use of adult norms
and extrapolations from these norms in the valuation of test
results from young patients.

Finally, our current and future studies of masking and
environmental noise will increasingly address issues relevant
to the physical and mental health of children. Studies of
non-human species have shown that exposure to high noise
levels results in greater anatomical and physiological injurie

f the inner ear of young compared to older animals (Falk et
l., 1974; Price, 1972). Although comparable human data are
ot available, it is possible that there may be similar age-
elated effects, with early periods of greater susceptibility.
ndeed, high noise levels in the home have been linked to
eficits in auditory discrimination, general listening skills,
arious language-related skills, and academic achievement
Cohen et al., 1972; Mills, 1975). This dimension of our
esearch should lend insight into noise levels that are appro-
riate for young children, pinpointing levels of long-term
xposure that lead to sensory deficits.

REFERENCES

ench, J., Collyer, J., Mentz, L., and Wilson, I. "Studies in
infant behavioral audiometry: II. Six-week-old infants"
Audiology 15:302-314, 1976.

ull, D., Schneider, B.A. and Trehub, S.E. "The masking of
octave-band noise by broad-spectrum noise: A comparison
of infant and adult thresholds" Perception and Psychophysics 30:101-106, 1981.

ull, D., Trehub, S.E. and Schneider, B.A. "A procedure for
infant psychophysical testing" (In preparation).

ohen, S., Glass, D.C. and Singer, J.E. "Apartment noise,
auditory discrimination and reading ability in children"
Journal of Experimental Social Psychology 9:407-422,
1973.

olburn, H.S. and Durlach, N.I. "Models of binaural inter-
action" in Carterette, E.C. and Friedman, M.P. (eds.)
Handbook of Perception, Vol. IV: Hearing (New York:
Academic Press), 1978.

rowell, D.H., Jones, R.H., Nakagawa, J.K. and Kapuniai, L.E.
"Heart rate response of human newborns to modulated pure
tones" Proceedings of the Royal Society of Medicine
64:474-474, 1971.

urlach, N.I. and Colburn, H.S. "Binaural and spatial hearing"
in Carterette, E.C. and Friedman, M.P. (eds.) Handbook
of Perception, Vol. IV: Hearing (New York: Academic
Press), 1978.

Elliott, L.L. "Performance of children aged 9 to 17 years on a test of speech intelligiblity in noise using sentence material with controlled work predictability" Journal of the Acoustical Society of America 66:651-653, 1979.

Engel, R. and Young, N.B. "Calibrated pure tone audiograms in normal neonates based on evoked electroencephalic responses" Neuropadiatrie 1:149-160, 1969.

Falk, S.A., Cook, R.O., Haseman, J.K. and Sanders, G.M. "Noise-induced inner ear damage in newborn and adult guinea pigs" Laryngoscope (April): 444-453, 1974.

Falk, S.A. and Farmer, J.C. "Incubator noise and possible deafness" Archives of Otolaryngology 97:385-387, 1973.

Hawkins, J.E., Jr. and Stevens, S.S. The masking of pure tones and of speech by white noise. Journal of the Acoustical Society of America 22,6-13, 1950.

Hutt, S.J., Hutt, C., Lenard, H.G., von Bernuth, H. and Muntjewerff, W.J. "Auditory responsivity in the human neonate" Nature 218:888-890, 1968.

Mills, J.H. "Noise and children: A review of literature" Journal of the Acoustical Society of America 58:767-779, 1975.

Moore, J.M., Thompson, G. and Thompson, M. "Auditory localization of infants as a function of reinforcement conditions" Journal of Speech and Hearing Research 40:29-34, 1975.

Price, G.R. "Loss in cochlear microphonic sensitivity in young cat ears exposed to intense sound" Journal of the Acoustical Society of America 51:104(a), 1972.

Peltzman, P., Kitterman, J.A., Ostwald, P.F., Manchester, D. and Heath, L. "Effects of incubator noise on human hearing" Journal of Auditory Research 10:335-339, 1970.

Schneider, B.A., Trehub, S.E. and Bull, D. "The development of basic auditory processes in infants" Canadian Journal of Psychology 33:306-319, 1979.

Schulman, C.A. and Wade, G. "The use of heart rate in the audiological evaluation of nonverbal children. Part II.

Clinical trials on an infant population" Neuropadiatrie 2:197-205, 1970.

Taylor, M.M. and Creelman, C.D. "PEST: efficient estimates of probability functions" Journal of the Acoustical Society of America 41:782-787, 1967.

Thompson, G. and Weber, B.A. "Responses of infants and young children to behavior observation audiometry" Journal of Speech and Hearing Research 39:140-147, 1974.

Trehub, S.E., Bull, D. and Schneider, B.A. "Infants' detection of speech in noise" Journal of Speech and Hearing Research 24:202-206, 1981(a).

Trehub, S.E., Bull, D. and Schneider, B.A. "Infant speech and nonspeech perception: A review of re-evaluation" in Schiefelbusch, R.L. and Bricker, D. (eds.) Early Language: Acquisition and Intervention (Baltimore: University Park Press), 1981(b).

Trehub, S.E., Schneider, B.A. and Bull, D. "Effect of reinforcement on infants' performance in an auditory detection task" Developmental Psychology 17:872-877, 1981.

Trehub, S.E., Schneider, B.A. and Endman, M. "Developmental changes in infants' sensitivity to octave-band noises" Journal of Experimental Child Psychology 29:282-293, 1980.

Wilson, W.R. "Assessment of auditory abilities in infants" in Minifie, F.D. and Lloyd, L.L. (eds.) Communicative and Cognitive Abilities: Early Behavioral Assessment (Baltimore: University Park Press), 1978.

Wilson, W.R. "Auditory behavior in infancy" in Gerber, S.E. and Mencher, G.T. (eds.) The Development of Auditory Behavior (New York: Grune & Stratton, Inc.), this volume.

THE PERCEPTION OF SPEECH
IN EARLY INFANCY: FOUR PHENOMENA

Patricia K. Kuhl
University of Washington, Seattle, WA

INTRODUCTION

It is just over ten years since the first experiment on
the perception of speech by young infants was published
(Eimas et al., 1971). In that time period, many studies on
infant speech perception have been completed and several comprehensive reviews of that literature have appeared (Eimas
and Tartier, 1979; Kuhl, 1979a; Jusczyk, 1981; Aslin et al.,
in press; Kuhl, in press a). Rather than provide a broad
overview of the work that has been done, this chapter describes
four phenomena related to the perception of speech and sound
by infants under six months of age.

The four phenomena highlight the interest areas of the
field, and show how those interests have broadened towards
the end of its first decade. Initially, our interest in
infants stemmed directly from the impact of the data on
theories of adult speech perception. Studies were directed
at the replication of the perceptual phenomena demonstrated
by adults. Certain theories (e.g., the "Motor Theory" of
speech perception, see Liberman et al., 1967) predicted the
outcome of infant experiments; they argued that the effects
seen in adults might require experience listening to the
sounds being tested or experience in the production of the
sounds.

Thus, early experiments were aimed at determining the
age at which the infant's perceptual responses to speech
were (1) constrained by linguistic categories, and (2) whether
these effects depended upon experience. The first phenomenon,
the demonstration of the "categorical perception" of speech
by infants, published by Eimas et al. (1971), and the second
phenomenon, the demonstration that infants exhibit "perceptual constancy" for speech sound categories, published by
Kuhl (1979b), exemplify this point. Both experiments tested

the extent to which young infants responded to speech in a manner conducive to the organization of sound into linguistic categories. The data from these two experiments showed, first, that infants as young as one month of age exhibited certain constraints on their ability to discriminate; infants were less sensitive to interphonemic variation in sound than they were to intraphonemic variation in sound (Eimas et al., 1971). And second, these experiments showed that infants equate phonetically identical (but easily discriminable) speech sounds even when the sounds are produced in different speech contexts and spoken by different talkers in varying tones of voice (Kuhl, 1979b). Thus, infants appear to perceive speech signals in linguistically appropriate ways.

Experiments of the third phenomenon explore the nonlinguistic value of speech. These examine speech as a signal with social significance. Previous research has shown that the speech directed by caretakers toward infants ("Motherese") differs greatly from that typically produced when those same caretakers are addressing other adults (Snow and Ferguson, 1977). The third phenomenon described here relates to the young infant's auditory preference for these kinds of signals. Fernald (1981) demonstrated that the four-month-old infant prefers to listen to "Motherese" as opposed to adult-directed speech, when given a choice. Moreover, the research shows that certain acoustic parameters,such as the fundamental frequency contours of the two types of utterances, are in themselves sufficient to obtain the preference for "Motherese" (Fernald and Kuhl, 1981). These data show, then, that the infant's response to speech and sound is dictated not only by its linguistic significance but its social significance. This type of experiment represents an important extension of the research on speech for infants to questions beyond theoretical models of adult speech perception.

The fourth, and last, phenomenon I describe relates to the infant's cognitive representation of speech. This experiment (Kuhl and Meltzoff, 1982) demonstrates that 18-week-old infants detect the correspondence between aurally and visually presented speech information. It suggests that infants relate specific articulatory postures to their concommitant speech sounds. This finding has important implications for vocal learning in infants, since vocal learning depends on the infant's ability to recognize the correspondence between articulatory movements and their resulting auditory consequences.

These four phenomena - 1) categorical perception, 2) perceptual constancy, 3) auditory preference for "Motherese," and 4) the bimodal perception of speech - span the duration of the field's history. They include the first publication in infant speech perception (Eimas et al., 1971) and one published just this year (Kuhl and Meltzoff, 1982). The four utilize different methods, and therefore provide a good sample of the technique used to study perception in infants at or under six months of age.

I.   Categorical Perception

One of the most interesting phenomena uncovered in early research on adults was "categorical perception" (Studdert-Kennedy et al., 1970). Categorical perception is a condition in which a listener's ability to discriminate two stimuli is predicted by his ability to label them differently. To demonstrate categorical perception, then, two tasks were compared: 1) one in which the subject labels each of the stimuli from an acoustic continuum that manipulates an acoustic cue in small steps; and 2) one in which the subject attempts to discriminate pairs of stimuli taken from the con-tinuum. These pairs of stimuli can be said to be drawn from the same phonetic category or from different phonetic cate-gories, according to how the stimuli were labeled by adult listeners. Typically, when two speech stimuli from a computer-synthesized continuum are presented for discrimina-tion, the listener's performance is at chance for stimuli drawn from the same phonetic category (that is, for stimuli that were labeled similarly) and near perfect for stimuli drawn from different phonetic categories (that is, for stimuli that were labeled differently).

We will illustrate the case for a speech-sound continuum that ranges perceptually from [ba] to [pa] (Abramson and Lisker, 1970). The acoustic variable being manipulated along this continuum is "voice-onset-time" (VOT) (Lisker and Abram-son, 1964). Naturally produced voiced and voiceless stop consonants are distinguished by the timing of the onset of laryngeal vibration (voicing) relative to the release of the constriction in the supralaryngeal musculature. In voiced stops (/ba,da,ga/), the onset of voicing precedes the release of the articulatory constriction by some 5 to 40 ms, whereas in voiceless stops, the release of the articulatory constric-tion precedes the onset of voicing by more than 25-40 ms. The VOT value of a stimulus indicates the duration, in ms, of the separation between the "burst" that occurs at the release of the constriction and the onset of voicing.

When adult English listeners are asked to "label" as
[ba] or [pa] the synthetic stimuli from this continuum, the
boundary value (the 50% point on the identification function)
falls at approximately +22 ms VOT. When the same listeners
are tested in a discrimination task with pairs of stimuli that
are equally distant on the continuum, they show enhanced discriminability for stimuli that straddle the phonetic boundary,
and relatively poor discriminability for stimuli that fall on
the same side of the boundary. In other words, they discriminate stimuli given different phonetic labels ([b] and [p])
very well, while failing to discriminate two stimuli given the
same phonetic label (either [b] or [p]). This produces a discrimination "peak" at the boundary between phonetic categories
as shown in Fig. 9-1. These are discrimination functions obtained from English-speaking adults. This non-monotonic discrimination function, labeled the "phoneme boundary effect" by
Wood (1976), was considered highly adaptive for the perception
of speech categories because it tended to highlight the between
category differences for speech stimuli while minimizing the
within-category differences.

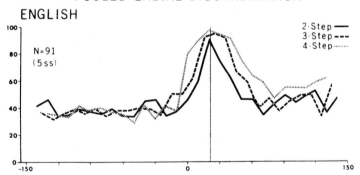

*Figure 9-1. Results of discrimination tests on English-
speaking adults. The continuum ranges from [ba] to [pa] (-150
ms VOT to +150 ms VOT). An "oddity" task was used in which
three stimuli were presented; two were identical and one was
different. The listener judged whether the "odd" stimulus
was in first, second, or third position. Two-, three-, and
four-step comparisons refer to 20-, 30-, and 40-ms differences between the stimulus pairs. In each case, a peak in
the discrimination function occurs near the phonetic boundary
(at approximately +25 ms) separating [ba] from [pa] (reprinted
from Abramson and Lisker, 1970).*

While we will not review its complete history here, the original view of categorical perception held that it was unique to the perception of speech sounds (Liberman et al., 1967). Since that time, a variety of non-speech signals that mimic the acoustic cues for speech sounds, and some visual stimuli as well, have been shown to produce similar effects (see Repp, in press, for a recent review). Moreover, it does not appear to be the case that the phenomenon for speech is unique to human listeners. Data show the "phoneme-boundary effect" is demonstrated by non-human mammals for a variety of phonetic contrasts (Kuhl, 1981; Kuhl and Padden, in press a; in press b). Nonetheless, while these data do not support the original notions concerning the exclusivity of the phenomenon (Studdert-Kennedy et al., 1970), there can be no doubt that it is highly conducive to the perception of phonetic categories. In fact, it has been argued (Kuhl and Miller, 1975; Kuhl, 1979) that the animal data support the notion that the acoustics of speech were designed to exploit certain features that were maximally discriminable by the mammalian auditory system. For the purposes of this discussion, we focus on the extent to which young infants demonstrate this set of perceptual constraints rather than debate the mechanisms hypothesized to underlie such constraints (see Kuhl, 1979c for further discussion). Our purpose, then, is to examine the extent to which infants, who cannot be asked to "label" a stimulus continuum, show evidence of differential discriminability for stimulus pairs on the continuum.

A method successfully used to study the infant's ability to discriminate speech-sound pairs is the high-amplitude-sucking (HAS) technique. Briefly, a speech sound is presented to the infant each time he produces a sucking response whose amplitude exceeds a criterion. That particular speech sound is presented until the infant's sucking rate drops below some decrement criterion (habituation). Then, experimental infants are presented with a different speech sound while control infants continue to be presented with the first sound.

The infant sucks on a blind nipple attached to a pressure transducer. The infant's sucking responses produce pressure changes inside the nipple that are monitored with a standard pressure transducer. An amplitude criterion is set for each infant during a "no-sound" baseline condition. After the baseline level has been established, a speech sound (typically 500 msec in duration) is presented immediately after each response with a maximum repetition rate of one per second. Typically, the infant's response rate increases and reaches a maximum. The same speech sound is presented until a 20 percent decrement in response rate occurs for two consecutive minutes. When this habituation criterion is met, infants in the experimental group are presented with a new sound while infants in the control group continue to hear the first sound. Both the experimental and the control infants are monitored for four minutes after the habituation criterion is met.

The mean response rate for the two minutes preceding the shift is subtracted from the mean response rate for the two minutes immediately following the shift to obtain a difference score for each infant. Experimental infants typically increase their response rates when the speech sound is changed (dishabituation) while control infants, who are presented with the same sound, either continue to decrease or do not change their response rates. A significant difference between the difference scores obtained by the two groups of infants is taken as evidence that the infants can discriminate the two speech sounds.

Eimas et al. (1971) tested one- and four-month-olds using the HAS technique and stimulus pairs drawn from the [ba-pa] continuum just described. They tested the discrimination of three pairs of stimuli, two within-category pairs (stimulus pairs in which both stimuli are labeled as either [ba] or [pa] by adults), and one between-category pair (stimulus pairs in which one stimulus was labeled [ba] and the other [pa] by adults). The two within-category stimulus pairs were -20 ms vs 0 ms VOT (both [ba]) and +60 ms vs +80 ms VOT (both [pa]). The between-category stimulus pair was +20 ms VOT vs +40 ms VOT ([ba] and [pa], respectively). For example, infants in the between-category group were presented with the +20 ms stimulus prior to the shift-point, and the +40 ms stimulus after the shift-point. In addition to these two experimental groups, another group of infants was tested as controls. They were not presented with a new sound at the shift point, but continued to hear the same sound.

Fig. 9-2 shows the results for the four-month-old infants. The number of criterion sucking responses is shown as a function of time for three groups of infants: 1) the between-category group, 2) the within-category group, and 3) the control group. In each case infants show a reliable increase by sucking responses after the baseline minute, followed by an eventual decline in the number of sucking responses (habituation). The infants in each of the three

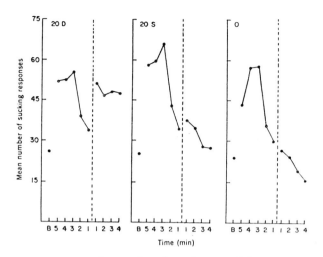

Figure 9-2. Mean number of criterion sucking responses as a function of time and experimental condition for the four-month-old infants. The dashed line indicates the shift point. The three experimental groups were (i) between-category (20D); (ii) within-category (20S); and (iii) control (0). Only the between-category group showed reliable sucking recovery (reprinted from Eimas et al., 1971).

groups responded similarly prior to the point of stimulus change. After the shift point, however, the three groups diverge. Only the between-category group provided evidence of a reliable increase in their sucking responses. Only this group appeared to discriminate the two stimuli. This pattern of response was similar for both one- and four-month-old infants.

Eimas et al.'s (1971) findings for stimuli from a [ba-pa] continuum were subsequently replicated for other speech stimuli. The infant's ability to discriminate between-category pairs, while failing to provide evidence of dis-criminating within-category pairs, was extended to a place-of-articulation continuum (/b-d-g/) by Eimas (1974) and to a speech continuum ranging from [ra] to [la] by Eimas (1975).

While these experiments on infants employed far fewer stimulus pairs in their discrimination tests than the number typically employed in speech experiments on adults, the data strongly suggest that infants under four months of age

demonstrate the "phoneme boundary effect." While we would
hesitate to say, given the difficulty of interpreting negative results, that infants are not capable of discriminating
within-category contrasts (adults can discriminate them under
certain testing conditions, see Carney et al., 1977), we can
say that they demonstrate enhanced discriminability for pairs
that are phonetically contrastive.

Regardless of the eventual determination of the mechanisms that underlie this phenomenon in young infants, be it
attributable to speech-specific mechanisms or to a more
general set of auditory predispositions (see Eimas and Tar-
ter, 1979, and Kuhl, 1970c, for discussion), this tendency
to partition a speech-sound continuum in a linguistically
relevant way has functional significance for the infant.

II. Perceptual Constancy for Speech-Sound Categories

The second phenomenon I describe also relates to the
infant's perceptual organization of speech. But rather than
focusing on the infant's ability to detect differences
between sounds, this phenomenon relates to the infant's perception of the similarities among sounds. Infants' data are
important here because many studies have demonstrated that
the acoustic cues critical to the perception of phonetic
units are altered by 1) their phonetic context, 2) the
talker who produces them, 3) their position in an utterance,
and 4) the rate at which they are spoken (see Liberman et
al., 1967, and Miller, 1981, for examples). This context-
specific variation is large enough that a set of acoustic
cues that are "invariant" across context, talker, position,
and rate has not been identified for most phonetic categories.
A listener's classification of speech in the absence of such
acoustically invariant cues has been related to the classic
cases of "constancy" in vision (Shankweiler et al., 1977;
Kuhl, 1976, 1979, 1980, in press b). In both instances,
perceivers recognize the identity of an event despite radical
transformations in its physical representation (see Kuhl, in
press c, for further discussion). Data demonstrating the age
at which infants recognize the phonetic equivalence among
auditory events provide evidence concerning the extent to
which a learning approach to the perception of constancy is
plausible.

Testing infants on a "perceptual constancy" task, as
opposed to the categorical perception case just reviewed,

requires a different set of stimuli and a different kind of
response from the infant. In the latter case, the stimuli
were computer synthesized and acoustic cues sufficient to
distinguish two phonetic categories were varied in step-wise
fashion to create a continuum. All other acoustic parameters
were held constant. The stimuli, then, sound very similar
and one is testing the degree to which the infant is sensitive to small variations in the critical acoustic variables
when they are isolated from other acoustic differences in the
stimuli. Conversely, in tests of constancy, certain dimensions, such as the phonetic context or talker, are purposely
varied. This has two results: 1) the values of the critical
dimensions underlying the perception of the target unit are
altered, and 2) additional dimensions that are acoustically
prominent, but irrelevant to the task of phonetic categorization, are introduced. For example, in the test of perceptual
constancy for vowels described below, the talker producing
the vowel is varied as well as the pitch contour of the
voice. Varying the talker not only alters the critical
acoustic cues underlying vowel identity (the formant frequencies), but introduces "timbre" differences inherent in
the speech of different talkers. These latter acoustic
variations, as well as the variations in pitch contour, can
be viewed as potential distractors for the infant. What we
want to know is whether the infant perceives the similarity
among these discriminably different instances of a particular
phonetic unit.

   The response required from the infant in tests of constancy differs from that required in tests of categorical
perception. In the latter, we are most interested in the
infant's perception of a difference. Thus, a change in the
response (sucking in this case) is evoked if the infant
detects a difference between the two stimuli. In the constancy case, we are most interested in the infant's perception of equivalence. We therefore arrange the test situation
such that a response (head-turning, as described below) is
evoked when the infant perceives the similarity among different instances.

   To achieve these goals, Kuhl (1979b) adapted a head-turn
technique, originally developed for assessing auditory
thresholds (Wilson et al., 1976), to test constancy. The
adaptation involved the use of a classic transfer-of-
learning design to determine whether an infant, trained to
discriminate a single token from one phonetic category from
a single token of a different phonetic category, would

demonstrate transfer-of-learning to a set of novel exemplars
from those categories.

The technique involved training 5.5- to 6.5-month-old
infants to make a head-turn response whenever a sound (for
example, /a/), repeated once every two seconds as a "background" stimulus, was changed to another sound, the "comparison" stimulus (for example, /i/), also repeated once every
two seconds for a period of six seconds. Head-turn responses
during the presentation of the comparison stimulus were rewarded with the presentation of a visual stimulus (an animated
toy animal). A comparison of the number of head-turn responses during these "change" trials with the number of head-turn
responses occurring during equally probable "control" trials
constituted the measure of the infant's performance. During
control trials, head-turn responses were monitored for an
identical observation interval but no change in the stimulus
occurred. Once a criterion level of performance on two individual tokens (one representing each of two categories) was
achieved, novel tokens were added to both the background and
the comparison categories, and transfer-of-learning from the
initial training tokens to novel exemplars was assessed.

Table 9-1 describes the stimuli in the background category and in the comparison category for each of five stages
in the first constancy experiment, one examining perception
of the vowels /a/ and /i/ (Kuhl, 1979b). In each category,
the number of vowels was increased until the two ensembles
contained six stimuli spoken by three different talkers
(male, female, and child) each with two different pitch
contours (rise and rise-fall). In the initial training
stage of the experiment, each of the two categories was
represented by a single token; these two tokens were matched
in every detail except for the critical cues which differentiate the two categories. In stage two, the pitch contour
of the vowels in both categories was randomly changed from
rise to rise-fall. In stage three, the talker producing the
vowels was randomly varied between the male voice and the
female voice. In stage four, both talkers produced the
vowels with a randomly-changing pitch contour. In the final
stage, the child's voice, also with pitch contour variations,
was added to the ensemble bringing the total number of tokens
in each category to six (3 talkers x 2 pitch contours).

Kuhl (1979b; in press b) examined two variations on the
transfer-of-learning design; the first involved a progressive
step-wise introduction of the novel tokens. The second

Table 9-1. The Stimulus Ensembles for the Background and Comparison Categories for All Five Stages of the /a/ vs. /i/ Experiment. The Talker and Pitch Contour Values for Each Stimulus Are Given in Parentheses (from Kuhl, 1979b).

	Experimental Stages	
	Background	Comparison
Conditioning	/a/ (Male, fall)	/i/ (Male, fall)
Initial training	/a/ (Male, fall)	/i/ (Male, fall)
Pitch variation	/a/ (Male, fall)	/i/ (Male, fall)
	/a/ (Male, rise)	/i/ (Male, rise)
Talker variation	/a/ (Male, fall)	/i/ (Male, fall)
	/a/ (Female, fall)	/i/ (Female, fall)
Talker X pitch variation	/a/ (Male, fall)	/i/ (Male, fall)
	/a/ (Male, rise)	/i/ (Male, rise)
	/a/ (Female, fall)	/i/ (Female, fall)
	/a/ (Female, rise)	/i/ (Female, rise)
Entire ensemble	/a/ (Male, fall)	/i/ (Male, fall)
	/a/ (Male, rise)	/i/ (Male, rise)
	/a/ (Female, fall)	/i/ (Female, fall)
	/a/ (Female, rise)	/i/ (Female, rise)
	/a/ (Child, fall)	/i/ (Child, fall)
	/a/ (Child, rise)	/i/ (Child, rise)

involved the immediate introduction, after initial training,
of all of the novel tokens. In the progressive transfer-of-
learning task, infants were tested at each of the five stages
in the experiment until they met a performance criterion,
and a trial-to-criterion measure was used to describe performance. In the immediate transfer-of-learning task, infants
were given a pre-set number of trials (equally probable change
and control) and an overall percent-correct measure on each o
the novel tokens was obtained.

The results of the progressive experiment on the [a-i]
contrast showed that infants demonstrated excellent transfer-
of-learning to the novel tokens. Most infants met the performance criterion in the minimum number of trials necessary.
More convincingly, however, in the immediate transfer-of-
learning experiment, performance was significantly above
chance on each of the novel tokens on the first trial during
which it was presented. Thus, the infants' responses could
not be attributed to training. The percentage of head-turn
responses to each of the tokens produced by individual
infants for all change trials during the transfer-of-learning
phase are shown in Fig. 9-3. As demonstrated, performance
was typically above 70% correct. For nearly half of the
infants, performance was nearly perfect.

These results have been extended to other more spectrally similar categories such as /a/ vs. /ɔ/ (Kuhl, in press
b), and to a variety of consonant categories (Kuhl, 1980;
Hillenbrand, 1980). In each case, the data provide strong
support for the notion that six-month-old infants recognize
auditory equivalence classes that conform to phonetic categories. That is to say, they appear to be able to "sort"
stimuli based on their phonetic identities.

The fact that infants perceive the similarities among
phonetically equivalent sounds, taken together with the
results suggesting that infants are differentially sensitive
to stimulus changes in the boundary regions between phonetic
categories, suggests that infants are well prepared for the
task of language learning. That they exhibit these tendencies
at such an early age, prior to a time that one could convincingly argue that they have "learned" to associate the different exemplars from a category, or to differentially discriminate synthetic exemplars, suggests that the mechanisms
responsible may be present at birth. Whether these mechanisms
will eventually be shown to be language-specific or not (see
Kuhl, 1979c for discussion), the infant's perceptual organization of speech is highly sophisticated by six months of age.

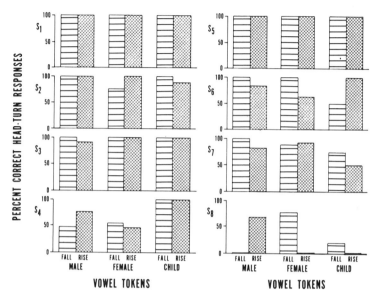

*Figure 9-3. Individual-subject data showing the generaliza-
tion of head-turn responses from the training token (Male-
fall) to novel instances of vowels spoken by female and child
talkers, with varying intonation contours (reprinted from
Kuhl, 1979b).*

It is also important to note, for the perceptual constancy demonstration just received, that the infant's tendency
to recognize the similarity among exemplars produced by
different talkers is of considerable importance to the development of speech production. It would be impossible for the
infant (due to constraints of vocal-tract anatomy and the
resulting acoustics) to learn to produce speech if the infant
adopted the strategy of trying to imitate the absolute formant frequencies; fundamental frequencies, or any other
relevant acoustic features produced by adult speakers.
Infants are simply not capable of reproducing the absolute
acoustic cues produced by the adult's vocal tract. Studies
like this particular one, demonstrating that infants readily
perceive equivalence in the vowels produced by men, women,
and children, suggest that the infant has an alternate
strategy available. If the infant recognizes the similarity
among tokens produced by a man, a woman, and a child, then it

seems likely that the infant recognizes the perceptual similarity between sounds produced by his/her own vocal tract and
those produced by a caretaker. If so, then the infant's
imitative attempts are guided by this perceptual match rather
than by any attempt to reproduce any of the absolute acoustic
features that adult talkers produce. The solution of this
"constancy" problem is thus an essential prerequisite for
vocal imitation.

III.   Infants Prefer to Listen to "Motherese"

     Research has demonstrated that the speech directed
toward young infants by adults is considerably simplified in
its syntactic form and semantic content (see Snow and Ferguson, 1977 for review) when compared to that directed toward
adults. This modification of the speech directed toward
infants has been termed "Motherese." Recent research on the
acoustic aspects of "Motherese" shows that it involves the
use of a higher overall fundamental frequency, exaggerated
intonation contours, and a slower tempo (Fernald and Simon,
in preparation). This alteration of the linguistic and pro-
sodic aspects of the speech directed towards infants is
apparently universal, having been reported to occur in
numerous languages (Ferguson, 1964).

     However extensive the data on a caretaker's tendency to
produce "Motherese" and detailed the arguments about the
potential effects of these kinds of acoustic signals on
infants (Stern, 1977), studies have not been directed toward
demonstrating the significance of these speech patterns for
infants. At the simplest level, studies have not attempted
to examine the extent to which the infant discriminates
"Motherese" from other kinds of speech. None has been
directed toward the infant's potential "preference" for
these speech patterns.

     In the experiments described here, these issues are
addressed. The studies test two hypotheses 1) that infants
demonstrate a preference for "Motherese" when presented with
a choice between infant-directed and adult-directed speech
("preference" is operationally defined as a stronger tendency
to make a head-turn response in the direction of one of two
alternative sound sources), and 2) to evaluate the contribution of selected acoustic parameters, such as fundamental
frequency, amplitude, and temporal organization, as determinants of this preference.

Fernald (1981) developed a technique to test the auditory preferences of four-month-olds. Briefly, infants sat on a parent's lap, facing a three-sided enclosure. Two loudspeakers were mounted in the right and left panels of the enclosure. The experiment was designed to give the infant a choice between listening to infant-directed and adult-directed speech. Head-turns to one side or the other determined which of the two kinds of signals the infant was presented with. For half of the infants, "Motherese" was presented following right head-turns while adult-directed speech was presented following left head-turns. For the other half of the infants, this left-right positioning was reversed.

The stimuli consisted of the speech of ten adult women, recorded as they talked to their four-month-olds and to an adult. None of the infants of these ten women participated in the experiment. One phrase was excerpted from the infant- and adult-directed utterances of each of the talkers. They were dubbed onto two separate channels of a tape recorder. Each phrase was approximately 8 seconds long.

These eight speech samples (4 talkers x 2 types) were acoustically analyzed to determine their fundamental frequency contours, their amplitude characteristics, and their durational characteristics. Figure 9-4 displays two of these features, their fundamental frequency ("pitch") contours, and durational characteristics. In three follow-up experiments, these acoustic characteristics were isolated. For example, in a second experiment, the two types of speech samples were represented by pure tones that followed the fundamental frequency characteristics of the speech samples (as shown in Fig. 9-4). The signals were presented at a constant amplitude, but were designed to follow the original signal's temporal characteristics. In a third experiment, the pure-tone signals were designed to follow the exact amplitude characteristics of the signals, while holding frequency constant. Again, these signals followed the durational characteristics of the original signals. Since these latter two experiments did not allow the separation of frequency (Experiment 2) or amplitude (Experiment 3) from temporal patterning, a fourth experiment was designed to examine the effect of these temporal characteristics in isolation. In this experiment, the pure-tone signals were of constant frequency and amplitude. The tones simply followed the on-off characteristics of the original signals.

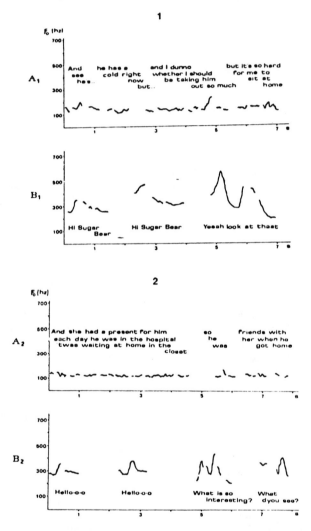

Figure 9-4. *Intonation contours from the speech of four women under two conditions: (A) adult-directed speech; (B) infant-directed speech "Motherese" (reprinted from Fernald, 1982).*

3

F_0 (hz)

A₃

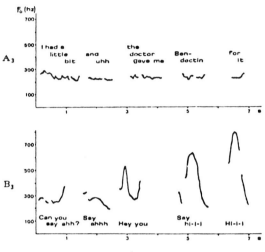

B₃

4

F_0 (hz)

A₄

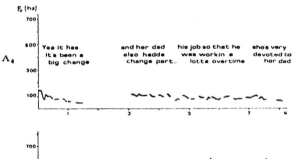

B₄

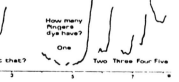

The procedure used in each of the four experiments involved familiarizing the infants, in counterbalanced order, with the signals presented from their left and right sides. Then, each infant was tested until 15 head-turn responses occurred. Each head-turn response was reinforced with the presentation of an 8-sec sample of either an infant- or adult-directed sample, depending on the direction of the turn.

The measure of the infant's performance was the total number of trials, out of 15, that the infant turned in the direction required to produce "motherese." These data were examined, using a variety of measures, to determine whether infants produced significantly more head-turns in the direction required to produce the infant-directed speech in the four experiments.

In the first experiment, where the two types of samples were represented by the original recordings of infant- and adult-directed speech, 33 of the 48 infants turned more often towards "Motherese" than towards adult-directed speech. This is significantly different from chance (p < .01 by binomial test). Group measures contrasting the total number of head-turns towards the two types of signals also produced significant results.

These data are displayed in Fig. 9-5. This graph also shows the percentage of infants who preferred the signals representing "Motherese" over adult-directed speech in Experiments 2, 3, and 4. As shown, the infant's preference for "Motherese" was maintained only in Experiment 2, when the two types of signals were represented by their fundamental frequency contours. In Experiments 3 and 4, when the signals differed only in the amplitude of the fundamental frequency, or only in the temporal (on-off) characteristics of the signals (with frequency and amplitude held constant), no significant difference was obtained.

The results of these experiments demonstrate 1) that infants given a choice will prefer to listen to "Motherese", and 2) that this preference is preserved when the signals are represented only by their fundamental frequency variations. The results suggest that one of the more compelling differences between infant-directed and adult-directed speech, that is, their fundamental frequency differences, may be a highly salient auditory characteristic for infants. These glissando-like melodic sequences have both a higher absolute frequency as well as an extended range. Which of these two

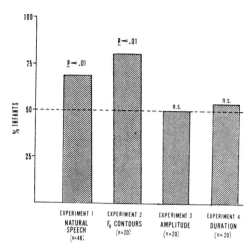

Figure 9-5. Percentage of infants producing a greater number of head-turn responses in the direction required to produce "Motherese" as opposed to Adult-directed speech in four experiments (reprinted from Fernald, 1982).

characteristics is primarily responsible for the infant's preference cannot be specified, since in Experiment 2, these two aspects of the fundamental frequency contours were confounded. Further research will need to be directed at the independent effects of pitch movement, per se, vs. absolute pitch, as determinants of auditory preference. The sequences of infant-directed speech were also more variable when compared to the adult-directed speech samples, so it is possible that this greater variability attracted the infant's attention. The exaggerated pitch range employed by mothers speaking to their infants specifically allows this greater variability. This may be one of the most compelling characteristics of "Motherese".

"Motherese" may serve the purpose of directing the infant's attention toward caretakers, as well as potentially serving to identify the infant's own mother. Research has suggested that newborn infants recognize and prefer their own mother's voices (DeCasper and Fifer, 1980). This may be due, in part, to experience "in utero," since recordings have shown that sounds below 1000 Hz are transmitted through the amniotic sac with little attenuation (Armitage et al., 1980). These studies on discrimination and preference for

voices, particularly those isolating the characteristics
typical of "Motherese" in general, and of the infant's own
mother, represent an important new extension of the kinds of
questions addressed to understand infants. This more socially
directed research should provide a more complete account of
the infant's use of audition to relate to his environment.

IV.   The Bi-modal Perception of Speech

     The impact of visual information on speech perception
has been well established in experiments on hearing-impaired
and normal adult populations (Erber, 1972; 1975; McGurk and
MacDonald, 1976; Summerfield, 1979). These studies have shown
that when auditory information is restricted - either naturally as it is for hearing-impaired listeners, or artificially
as in laboratory experiments on lip-reading - the visual information provided by watching a talker's mouth movements
significantly improves the perception of speech.

     Recent data on normal-hearing adults reveals another
related phenomenon. Research shows that when auditory information is not degraded in any way but is presented simultaneously with visual information that does not agree with that
presented acoustically, illusory percepts can result (McGurk
and MacDonald, 1976; Summerfield, 1979). That is, the perceiver reports a syllable that was presented neither to the
visual modality nor to the auditory modality. Interestingly,
even though this information is discrepant and picked up by
two different modalities, the perceiver experiences a pheno-
menally unified and coherent percept of a single talker and
a single message. Theoretical accounts of this phenomenon
recognize that information about speech entering the two
modalities must be co-registered in a common metric in order
for this to occur. Thus, speech information in adults, at
some level, must be represented bi-modally.

     An examination of the impact of visually presented infor-
mation on speech perception in infants could potentially contribute to our understanding of the infant's mastery of
auditory-articulatory relations. Lip-reading phenomena in
adults imply that perceivers relate specific articulatory
postures to their concommitant speech sounds. Such examples
of the adults' "knowledge" of the relationship between audition and articulation is perhaps not surprising, since the
adult is a practiced speaker. However, it is precisely this
relationship between articulatory movements and their auditory

correlates that the infant must presumably learn. The eventual mastery of a set of rules concerning this auditory-
articulatory mapping allows the child to reproduce, at will,
a particular sound with his/her own articulators. While
theorists have speculated that infant "babbling" serves to
teach the infant the rules relating articulatory movements
to sound (Studdert-Kennedy, 1976; Kent, 1980; Netsell, 1980),
no empirical data exist that provide information concerning
the development of the recognition of this relationship.

One way to pose the auditory-articulatory mapping problem
to infants is to examine the degree to which the infant recognizes the correspondence between a particular articulatory
gesture, presented visually, and a particular sound, presented
acoustically; in other words, to pose a lip-reading problem
to infants. In the experiment reported next (Kuhl and
Meltzoff, 1982), infants were tested in a visual paired-
comparison technique in which the infant was shown two identical faces producing, in synchrony, two different vowel
sounds. A single sound that matched only one of the two faces
was acoustically presented through a loudspeaker located midway between the two faces. The hypothesis was that, if
infants were capable of detecting the correspondence between
the acoustically and visually presented speech information,
they would look significantly longer at the face that
"matched" the sound rather than at the "mismatched" face;
if they did not, they would devote an equal amount of time
looking at each face.

The technique used to test this hypothesis was one previously used to study cross-modal perception in infancy
(Meltzoff and Borton, 1979). The infants were shown two
filmed images side by side of a talker articulating, in synchrony, two different vowel sounds (Fig. 9-6). The sound
track corresponding to one of the two faces was presented
through a loudspeaker directly behind the screen and midway
between the visual images. The visual stimuli consisted of
two 16 mm film loops, each containing a repeated sequence of
ten /a/ vowels and ten /i/ vowels. The articulations were
produced once every three seconds by the same female talker.
One film loop displayed them in the reverse orientation. The
acoustic stimuli were 16 mm sound tracks containing the
sequences of /a/'s and /i/'s that the talker produced while
being filmed. Either the /a/ or /i/ sound track could be
played with either film loop. The stimuli were carefully
produced such that their durations fell within a narrowly
constrained range; and this, together with the procedure used

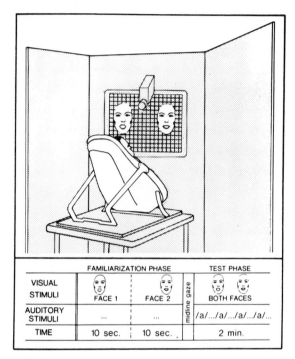

Figure 9-6. *The experimental apparatus and procedure used in the bimodal speech perception experiment.* *The infants were shown two facial displays of the same female talker, one articulating the vowel /a/ and the other articulating the vowel /i/.* *The sound track corresponding to one of the two faces was presented through a loudspeaker placed behind the screen midway between the faces (reprinted from Kuhl and Meltzoff, 1982).*

to align the sound and film tracks, assured that each sound track was temporally synchronized to both faces equally well.

The experimental procedure involved a familiarization phase and test phase (Fig. 9-6). During the familiarization phase, an infant was shown each face separately for 10 sec without sound. Following this 20-sec period, the faces were briefly covered until the infant's gaze returned to midline. Then, the sound was turned on and both faces were presented for the 2-minute test phase. The sound presented to the infants, the left-right positioning of the two faces, the

order of familiarization, and the sex of the infant were
counterbalanced. Thirty-two infants between 18- and 20-weeks
of age were tested.

Infants were placed in an infant seat within a three-
sided cubicle, 46 cm from the two facial displays. The
faces were life-size and their centers were separated by 38
cm. The only source of visible light in the room was that
provided by the films themselves. An infrared camera posi-
tioned between the two faces provided a recording of the
infant's face allowing an observer to record the amount of
time the infant spent fixating the left and right facial
images. The fixations were scored from videotape by an independent observer who could neither hear the sound nor see
the faces presented to the infant.

The results of the experiment clearly demonstrated that
the identity of the acoustically presented vowel systemati-
cally influenced the infants' visual fixations. The percentage of total fixation time devoted to the matched vs. mismatched face was calculated for each infant. Twenty-four of
the 32 infants looked longer at the face matching the sound
than at the mismatched face ($p < .01$, binomial test). The
mean percentage fixation time devoted to the matching face
by the group was 73.63%, which is significantly different
from the 50% chance level ($t = 4.67$, $p < .001$). There were
no significant left-right preferences, face preferences, or
familiarization order effects.

In a second experiment, Kuhl and Meltzoff (1982) made
an initial attempt to specify the nature of the auditory
information that was critical to the detection of these
auditory-visual correspondences. They altered the original
acoustic stimuli (the sets of /a/ and /i/ vowels) so as to
remove the spectral information necessary to identify the
vowels (formant frequencies) while preserving their temporal
characteristics (amplitude and duration). The stimuli were
computer-generated pure-tone signals centered at the average
fundamental frequency of the female talker (200 Hz), whose
onset and offset characteristics and overall amplitude enve-
lopes were synthesized to duplicate those of the original
vowels. If infants based their detection of these auditory-
visual correspondences on their knowledge of the relationship
between a particular articulatory movement and its concomi-
tant speech sound, then the acoustic information provided the
infant must be sufficient to identify the speech sound.
These signals did not contain such information, so the effect
should not be obtained.

Conversely, Kuhl and Meltzoff (1982) argued that
this experiment served as a test of an alternative hypothesis, namely that infants in their first experiment were
not relying on spectral information, but on temporal
information to link particular face-voice pairs. While
Kuhl and Meltzoff (1982) argued that the technique they
employed to align the sound and film tracks made such a
temporal hypothesis an unlikely explanation for the outcome
of their first experiment, the second experiment addressed
the issue directly. If infants in the first experiment were
relying on temporal information to link particular face-voice
pairs, then they should still look longer at the "matched"
face, even though it was represented only by its sine-wave
amplitude envelope. Alternatively, if the spectral information contained in the vowels was necessary for the detection of these auditory-visual correspondences, performance
should drop to chance.

Another group of 32 infants between 18 and 20 weeks was
tested using the exact same procedure and the new stimuli.
The results showed that the mean percent fixation time to
the "matched" face dropped to chance (54.6%, p <.40). Thus,
the data suggest that some aspect of the spectral information
is critical. Further experiments will be necessary to determine whether the detection of these correspondences requires
spectral information that allows the vowel to be identified,
or whether a signal that matches the vowel's spectral pattern
without specifying its identity is sufficient.

These findings suggest that infants recognize that particular speech sounds emanate from mouths moving in particular
ways. This fact has implications for social, cognitive, and
linguistic development. From a social perspective, this
highly specific ability may serve to direct the infant's
visual attention toward a speaker who is talking, and play
a role in the acquisition of vocal turn-taking (Stern et al.,
1975; Bruner, 1975). From the standpoint of cognitive development, these data add to a growing list of examples which
attest to the young infant's ability to detect intermodal
equivalences for information presented to different modalities
(Spelke, 1976, 1979; Meltzoff and Moore, 1977; Meltzoff and
Borton, 1979). These data suggest that infants are not limited
to the registration of sense-specific information. Rather, it
suggests that they are predisposed to represent information
intermodally (Meltzoff, 1981). This notion has potential

clinical implications for infants born with sensory deficits.
Data on adults confirm the fact that speech reception is
improved when the information provided by lip-reading is combined with spectral information delivered through a tactile
aid (Sparks et al., 1978). Perhaps infants born deaf (or
blind) could also be aided by the co-delivery of information
from two different sensory modalities.

The data are most relevant, however, to linguistic development. Detection of auditory-visual correspondences for
speech suggests that, by 18 weeks of age, the infant pos-
sesses some rather specific knowledge of the relationship
between the auditory and articulatory correlates of speech.
Such an ability may reflect specific associations that were
learned simply by watching caretakers speak. On the other
hand, this demonstration may reflect a more general intermodal representation of speech, one not limited to specific
associative pairings between speech information presented
acoustically and visually, but one that encompasses its
sensori-motor equivalents as well.

Kuhl and Meltzoff (1982) advocated the broader interpretation. They cited the fact that about a third of the infants
tested in their first experiment (who listened to the vowels),
but only one of those tested in their second experiment (who
listened to the non-speech signals), produced utterances
typical of "babbling." These infants appeared to be imita-
ting the female talker, mimicking the spectrum, duration, and
fundamental frequency contours of her vowels (see Kuhl and
Meltzoff, 1982 for examples). These findings suggest that
infants are 1) cognizant of auditory-motor equivalents, and
2) capable of directing their articulators to produce an
aurally specified target.

Moreover, other data suggest that infants are cognizant
of visual-motor equivalents. Meltzoff and Moore (1977) have
demonstrated that three-week-olds, and more recently that
neonates (Meltzoff and Moore, in press), imitate facial gestures such as mouth opening, tongue protrusion, and lip protrusion. Some of these gestures, such as the mouth-opening
gesture, are speech-like, and may be taken as support for the
idea that infants recognize visual-motor equivalents for
speech.

These demonstrations of complex auditory-motor and visual-
motor mappings, in combination with the demonstration of the
auditory-visual perception of speech, suggest that the broader

interpretation merits consideration. Future studies will aim
to specify the relationship between these auditory-visual
mappings and vocal imitation, and the extent to which either
or both depend on "babbling" or any other specific kind of
experience. This demonstration of the bimodal perception of
speech in 18-week-old infants represents a first step in
elucidating the nature of the mechanism responsible for vocal
learning in infancy.

SUMMARY

Four phenomena related to the infant's perception of
speech have been described. These demonstration experiments
attest to the fact that, by six months of age, the infant's
responses to speech are fairly sophisticated; and this has
important implications for linguistic, social, and cognitive
development.

From a linguistic perspective, the data show that the
infant's response to speech is not governed by arbitrary
divisions and/or groupings of stimuli, but that it conforms
to phonological categories. Infants show heightened sensitivity to stimulus differences when they mark the distinction
between phonetic categories. They show reduced sensitivity
to these same physical differences when they do not mark the
differences between phonetic categories.

Moreover, infants recognize the phonetic equivalence
among discriminably different instances representing phonetic
categories. In so doing, they show the ability to ignore
acoustically prominent but irrelevant features of the stimuli
Infants do not perceptually group these instances because the
fail to discriminate the differences between them. Rather,
they appear capable of selectively responding to a single
dimension that predicts phonetic identity and of "sorting"
the stimuli on that dimension. That a variety of "sorting
rules" are available to the infant is also clear given the
data (see Kuhl, 1980 for discussion).

While it is not possible at this stage to attribute these
linguistically adaptive responses to speech-specific processing mechanisms, there can be no doubt that they well serve
the language-learning infant. Debates about the nature and
origins of these phonemena do not and should not detract from
the recognition of their functional significance to the
infant.

While experiments examining the linguistic value of speech for infants have produced as interesting a theoretical puzzle as any in infant development, they have not addressed its non-linguistic significance for infants. Yet, for adults, speech communicates both linguistic and non-linguistic information. Studies on infants' sound preferences represent an initial attempt to study its non-linguistic significance for infants. Signals (like "Motherese") that are argued to 1) achieve and hold attention, 2) communicate positive affect, and 3) identify a group of people that help ensure survival, are particularly appropriate for these kinds of questions.

These studies indicated that fundamental frequency may be the primary determinant of a preference for "Motherese." Fundamental frequency carries two kinds of information; it imparts linguistic information such as sentential stress and the locations of major constituent boundaries, and it imparts information about the speaker's identity, affect, and intent. The study of its perception by infants may lead to an understanding of infants' abilities to derive different kinds of information from a single acoustic parameter. If so, these studies could contribute to a comprehensive theory of speech and sound perception in infancy.

A similar argument concerning the kinds of studies that will lead to a comprehensive theory of infant speech perception can be made for studies that examine the cognitive representation of speech in infants. The demonstration experiment involving the bimodal perception of speech had very specific implications for linguistic development. It was an attempt to examine the auditory-articulatory representation of speech; a representation, derived or inherent, that the infant must be cognizant of in order to learn to speak. Yet, it is this specific kind of linguistic question that requires a more comprehensive view of an infant's cognitive abilities. The problem necessitates an understanding of the infants' ability to represent information across modality and interface sensory and motor representations. The eventual explanation of vocal learning will require a theory that accounts for the infant's cognitive representation of action in terms of its sensory and motor equivalents. Whether studying these classic issues in cognitive development in the context of speech will lead to a theory that is speech-specific, or one that embraces (and elucidates in fine detail) the problem of sensori-motor mappings in a general way, remains to be seen.

REFERENCES

Abramson, A. and Lisker, L. "Discriminability along the voicing continuum: Cross-language tests," in Proceedings of the 6th International Congress of Phonetic Sciences (1967) (Prague: Academia), 1970.

Armitage, S., Baldwin, B., and Vince, M. "The fetal sound environment of sheep," Science 208: 1173-1174, 1980.

Aslin, R., Pisoni, D., and Jusczyk, P. "Auditory development and speech perception in infancy," in Mussen, P.H. (ed.) Carmichael's Handbook of Infant Development, in press.

Bruner, J. "From communication to language: A psychological perspective," Cognition 3: 255-287, 1975.

Carney, A., Widen, G., and Viemeister, N. "Noncategorical perception of stop consonants differing in VOT," Journal of the Acoustical Society of America 62: 961-970, 1977.

DeCasper, A. and Fifer, W. "Of human bonding: Newborns prefer their mothers' voices," Science 208:1174-1176, 1980.

Eimas, P. "Auditory and linguistic processing of cues for place of articulation by infants," Perception and Psychophysics 16: 513-521, 1974.

Eimas, P. "Auditory and phonetic coding of the cues for speech: Discrimination of the /r-l/ distinction by young infants," Perception and Psychophysics 18: 341-347, 1975.

Eimas, P., Siqueland, E., Jusczyk, P. and Vigorito, J. "Speech perception in infants," Science 171: 303-306, 1971.

Eimas, P. and Tartter, V. "On the development of speech perception: Mechanisms and analogies," in Reese, H. and Lipsitt, L. (eds.) Advances in Child Development and Behavior Vol. 13 (New York: Academic Press), 1979.

Erber, N. "Auditory, visual, and auditory-visual recognition of consonants by children with normal and impaired hearing," Journal of Speech and Hearing Research 2: 413-422, 1972.

Erber, N. "Auditory-visual perception of speech," Journal of Speech and Hearing Disorders 40: 481-492, 1975.

Ferguson, C. "Baby talk in six languages," American Anthropologist 66: 103-114, 1964.

Fernald, A. "Four-month-olds prefer to listen to 'Motherese'," presented at the Society for Research in Child Development, Boston, 1981.

Fernald, A. and Kuhl, P. "Fundamental frequency as an acoustic determinant of infant preference for 'Motherese'," presented at the Society for Research in Child Development, Boston, 1981.

Fernald, A. and Simon, T. "Expanded intonation contours in mothers' speech to newborns," in preparation.

Hillenbrand, J. Perceptual Organization of Speech Sounds by Young Infants, unpublished Ph.D. dissertation, University of Washington, 1980.

Jusczyk, P. "Infant speech perception: A critical appraisal," in Eimas, P. and Miller, J. (eds.) Perspectives on the Study of Speech (Hillsdale, NJ: Lawrence Erlbaum Assoc.), 1981.

Kent, R. "Articulatory-acoustic perspectives on speech development," in Stark, R. (ed.) Language Behavior in Infancy and Early Childhood (New York: Elsevier), 1980.

Kuhl, P. "Speech perception in early infancy: The acquisition of speech sound categories," in Hirsh, S., Eldredge, D., Hirsh, I., and Silverman, S. (eds.) Hearing and Davis: Essays Honoring Hallowell Davis (St. Louis: Washington University Press), 1976.

Kuhl, P. "The perception of speech in early infancy," in Lass, N. (ed.) Speech and Language: Advances in Basic Research and Practice (New York: Academic Press), 1979a.

Kuhl, P. "Speech perception in early infancy: Perceptual constancy for spectrally dissimilar vowel categories," Journal of the Acoustical Society of America 66: 1668-1679, 1979b.

Kuhl, P. "Models and mechanisms in speech perception: Species comparisons provide further contributions," Brain, Behavior Evolution 16: 374-408, 1979c.

Kuhl, P. "Perceptual constancy for speech-sound categories in early infancy," in Yeni-Komshian, G., Kavanagh, J., and Ferguson, C. (eds.) Child Phonology: Perception and Production (New York: Academic Press), 1980.

Kuhl, P. "Perception of speech and sound in early infancy," in Salapatek, P. and Cohen, L.B. (eds.) Handbook of Infant Perception (New York: Academic Press), in press.

Kuhl, P. "Perception of auditory equivalence classes for speech in early infancy," Infant Behavior and Development, in press.

Kuhl, P. "Constancy, categorization, and perceptual organization for speech and sound in early infancy," in Mehler, J. (ed.) Neonatal Cognition: Beyond the Blooming Confusion (Hillsdale, NJ: Lawrence Erlbaum Assoc.), in press.

Kuhl, P. and Meltzoff, A. "The bimodal perception of speech in infancy," Science, in press.

Kuhl, P. and Miller, J. "Speech perception in the chinchilla voiced-voiceless distinction in alveolar plosive consonants," Science 190: 69-72, 1975.

Kuhl, P. and Padden, D. "Speech discrimination by macaques: auditory constraints on the evolution of language," Perception and Psychophysics, in press a.

Kuhl, P. and Padden, D. "Speech discrimination by macaques: Enhanced discrimination at the phonetic boundaries between speech-sound categories," Journal of the Acoustical Society of America, in press b.

Liberman, A., Cooper, F., Shankweiler, D., and Studdert-Kennedy, M. "Perception of the speech code," Psychological Review 74: 431-461, 1967.

Lisker, L. and Abramson, A. "A cross-language study of voicing in initial stops: Acoustical measurements," Word 20: 384-422, 1964.

McGurk, K. and MacDonald, J. "Hearing lips and seeing voices," Nature 264: 746-748, 1976.

Meltzoff, A. "Imitation, intermodal coordination, and representation in early infancy," in Butterworth, G. (ed.) Infancy and Epistemology (London: Harvester Press), 1981.

Meltzoff, A. and Borton, T. "Intermodal matching by human neonates," Nature 282: 403-404, 1979.

Meltzoff, A. and Moore, K. "Imitation of facial and manual gestures by human neonates," Science 198: 75-78, 1977.

Meltzoff, A. and Moore, K. "Human newborns imitate adult facial gestures," Child Development, in press.

Miller, J. "Effects of speaking rate on segmental distinctions," in Eimas, P. and Miller, J. (eds.) Perspectives on the Study of Speech (Hillsdale, NJ: Lawrence Erlbaum Assoc.), 1981.

Netsell, R. "The acquisition of speech motor control: A perspective with directions for research," in Stark, R. (ed.) Language Behavior in Infancy and Early Childhood (New York: Elsevier), 1980.

Repp, B. "Categorical perception: Issues, methods, findings," in Lass, N. (ed.) Speech and Language: Advances in Basic Research and Practice (New York: Academic Press), in press.

Shankweiler, D., Strange, W., and Verbrugge, R. "Speech and the problem of perceptual constancy," in Shaw, R. and Bransford, J. (eds.), Perceiving, Acting and Knowing: Toward an Ecological Psychology (Cambridge: Cambridge University Press), 1977.

Snow, C. and Ferguson, C. Talking to Children: Language Input and Acquisition (Cambridge: Cambridge University Press), 1977.

Sparks, D., Kuhl, P., Edmonds, A., and Gray, G. "Investigating the MESA (Multipoint Electrotactile Speech Aid): The transmission of segmental features of speech," Journal of the Acoustical Society of America 63: 246-257, 1978.

Spelke, E. "Infants' intermodal perception of events,"
Cognitive Psychology 8: 553-560, 1976.

Spelke, E. "Perceiving bimodally specified events in
infancy," Developmental Psychology 15: 626-636, 1979.

Stern, D. The First Relationship: Mother and Infant (Cambridge: Harvard University Press), 1977.

Stern, D., Jaffe, J., Beebe, B., and Bennett, S. "Vocalizing
in unison and in alternation: Two modes of communication
in the mother-infant dyad," Annals of the New York
Academy of Sciences 263: 89-100, 1975.

Studdert-Kennedy, M., Liberman, A., Harris, K. and Cooper, F.
"Role of formant transitions in the voiced-voiceless
distinction for stops," Journal of the Acoustical
Society of America 55: 653-659, 1970.

Summerfield, Q. "Use of visual information for phonetic
perception," Phonetica 36: 314-331, 1979.

Wilson, W., Moore, J., and Thompson, G. "Auditory thresholds
of infants utilizing visual reinforcement audiometry
(VRA)," paper presented at the convention of the American
Speech and Hearing Association, Houston, 1976.

Wood, C. "Discriminability, response bias, and phoneme categories in discrimination of voice onset time," Journal
of the Acoustical Society of America, 60: 1381-1389,
1976.

Part III

Linguistic Development

INFANT BABBLING AS A MANIFESTATION
OF THE CAPACITY FOR SPEECH

D. Kimbrough Oller
University of Miami

Introduction

There has long been confusion concerning the nature of
the relationship between babbling of infants and mature
speech. While many empirical questions remain unanswered
concerning the relationship, a large proportion of what has
been written about infant vocalizations is based on unreason-
able assumptions that do not warrant empirical refutation.
Instead, they can be dismissed on the basis of common sense.

The primary source of the confusion is Jakobson's (1941)
widely cited discussion asserting that there is no phonetic
relationship between infant babbling and speech. The baby's
babbling sounds were viewed as a random assortment of sounds
from all the world's languages, each produced with equal ease,
while the sounds of early speech were seen as ordered and
regular, with a clear hierarchy of phonetic preferences. The
position was inspired by an apparent belief that the onset of
speech had certain maturational magic, and represented the
moment at which our uniquely human linguistic heritage
asserted itself. One might imagine the Jakobsonian infant
passing the great linguistic threshold and then never looking
back, for what lies behind is not his own history, but that
of some other kind of creature, the prelinguistic kind, the
kind that has no phonetics.

Although the onset of meaningful speech is a landmark
event in the maturation of the organism, it is unwarranted
to exclude examination of important developmental precursors
to the emergence of that speech capacity. The precursors can
be examined by investigation of the phonetic relationship
between meaningful speech and infant babbling of the pre-
meaningful period. Jakobson ruled out such a relationship
with his sweeping caveat and many members of the community
of scholars accepted his view for a generation. One outcome

of the acceptance has been a relative lack of active interest
in infant vocalizations and a tendency on the part of many to
assert that there is no purpose in empirically studying infant
vocal sounds since such study could, according to this view,
be of no use in the understanding of the speech capacity.

The key issue in exploding the Jakobsonian myth lies in
the common sense recognition that any sounds produced by any
vocal tract can be analogized within the framework of a minimally general theory of speech to the sounds of any other
vocal tract. If we wished to examine the phonetic relationship between the songs of the nightingale and the speech of
any human being, a sufficiently general theory of speech
could be employed as a framework for the comparison. Such
a task might have substantial interest, especially if it
provided comparison of timing for phrases and phrase components in the two cases, or investigated similarities in the
use of features such as rise time, pitch modulation, etc.

A minimally general theory of speech does not involve
any new creation but merely the naming of an implicit theory
that has been in the background of the educations of all who
are students of spoken language. The theory has been called
"metaphonology" or "metaphonetics" (Oller, 1978, 1980), and
for the present purposes there is no need to specify it more
fully than to say that it includes an account of the general
parameters from which phonologies construct their inventories
of concrete elements. Among the concrete elements are individual classes of consonants, vowels, stress values, intonation contours, etc. Among the parameters accounted for in
metaphonology are timing, amplitude, pitch, resonance, etc.
Clearly, any two vocal systems can be compared in terms of
metaphonological parameters, and by this means a phonetic
relationship between any two systems of vocalization can be
specified. It is clear then that there is a phonetic relationship between infant vocalizations and speech and that
furthermore, such a relationship must obtain given a general
theory of phonetic parameters.

Continuity, discontinuity, and relatedness

A number of treatments of babbling have focused on a
"continuity-discontinuity" controversy. Jakobson is credited
with having inspired a theory of discontinuity between sounds
of babbling and speech. Others, including me, have been
identified as supporting a theory of continuity between
sounds of babbling and speech. To the extent that the

presumed continuity theory emphasizes continuous development
of a speech capacity and allows possible changes in the
extent of similarity of babbling and speech across time, it
is a tenable theoretical stance. However, the implication
within a continuity theory that there are no important
phonetic differences between babbling and speech is theoretically unsound. To suggest that there is a relationship
between two vocal systems is to suggest that there are similarities, but it is not to deny that there are differences.
A full specification of the relationship of babbling and
speech should incorporate both a discussion of similarities
and differences as they are found. While it is possible that
differences will not be found in empirical studies, it is
unwise to prejudge the data.

The recognition that both similarities and differences
are possible in the empirical study of comparative developmental phonetics suggests a title other than "continuity
theory" for the theoretical position espoused here. A
"relatedness theory" seems appropriate since that phrase
would not imply similarity to the exclusion of difference.

Relatedness of late babbling and early meaningful speech

In addressing the empirical data on infant vocalizations,
one is immediately faced with substantial differences between
the kinds of vocalizations produced at early and late stages
of the first year of life. These differences impose different
theoretical requirements on attempts to describe the relationship of the infant sounds and mature speech. The goal of
description is always to provide a maximally enlightening
specification of the relationship. By the end of the first
year of life this specification is relatively straightforward
since, by that age, infants produce sounds that are much like
mature speech. The sounds include identifiable consonant-
like and vowel-like elements. One of the most interesting
approaches to comparison of these late babbling sounds and
meaningful speech was suggested by Lewis (1936) who simply
described some of the commonly occurring early words of child
speech and noted that they were composed of sounds and syllables that appeared to be common in infant babbling of the
period just before the onset of speech. Lewis' observation
was unquantified, but held in it the grain of a truth that
would emerge as a forest of observations by later scholars.

Menyuk (1968) provided a comparison of the frequency of
usage of various phonetic/phonological features in late

babbling and early meaningful speech. She commented in her
conclusions that the similarity of occurrence rates in the two
cases was striking. Cruttenden (1970) also provided a description of babbling and concluded that there seemed to be
great similarities of babbled sounds and early meaningful
speech. Many other studies have confirmed the observation
that, far from being unrelated, the sounds of babbling are
much like those of early speech in childhood (see e.g.,
Vanvik, 1971; Nakazima, 1962; Murai, 1963; de Boysson Bardies,
Sagart, and Bacri, 1981).

    The desire to quantify the relationship further led us
(Oller, Wieman, Doyle, and Ross, 1975) to consider the proportion of usage of various categories of speech or speech-
like sounds for which there was clear documentation of a
"preference" in the speech of early childhood. The term
"preference" does not here necessarily imply conscious
activity, but merely a systematic tendency of the child to
use a particular sound or sound sequence to the exclusion of
of in greater frequency than some other sound or sound
sequence. For example, in early child speech, it is well-
documented that single consonants are preferred over consonant
clusters (e.g., CV or VC syllables are preferred over CCV or
VCC syllables). When, for example, children try to produce
a sequence which in the adult form has a CCV shape, they tend
to produce a CV shape instead (stay > tay, true > tue, etc.).
The reverse (e.g., replacement of CV syllables with CCV types)
does not commonly occur. Consequently there is a higher proportion of syllables with singleton consonants in the speech
of young children than of syllables with consonant clusters.
Similarly initial consonants are more common in young child
speech than final consonants, initial stops are more common
than fricatives, initial unaspirated stops are more common
than aspirated ones, final voiceless obstruents are more
common than voiced ones, glides are more common than liquids,
apical consonants are more common than dorsal ones, and
fricatives and affricates are more common relative to stops
in final position than in initial position.

    These well-documented tendencies of early child speech
were examined in babbling. The babbling of 10 infants, five
infants six to eight months old, and five, eleven to twelve
months old, showed the same preferences that occurred in early
meaningful speech. The infants more commonly produced CV
syllables, initial consonants, initial stops, etc. In fact
the study showed extraordinary similarity of babbling and
early speech.

It can be concluded that a variety of studies of infant vocalizations shows that there is substantial similarity between late babbling and speech. Further the fact that infant sounds have much in common with speech, suggests the conclusion that babbling manifests the emergence of a phonological capacity.

Reliability of observations in studies of babbling

The above-cited studies indicating similarities of babbling and speech, on the whole, are based on phonetic transcription of infant and young child sounds. Critics of research on infant phonetics have attacked such methods, claiming that transcriptions of the sounds of infancy lack objectivity. Lynip (1951) claimed that transcription is not appropriate since "there is no international phonetic alphabet for a baby." The merit of Lynip's contention lies in the fact that, indeed, some sounds produced by babies do not seem very amenable to description in terms of the units of the International Phonetic Alphabet. That problem can be overcome, however, by supplementing and revising the phonetic description to incorporate idiosyncrasies of infant vocalizations. Ultimately, Lynip's position (denying the utility of transcription in studying babbling) is ill-conceived because transcription is necessary to delineate the relationship of babbling and speech. While instrumental analyses are useful, they cannot ultimately respond to the functional (and indeed "crucial") question of how well infant sounds could serve the purposes of speech communication.

To the extent that the babbling infant produces sounds that are similar to those of mature speakers of natural languages, the infant is approximating functionally useful sound types. The judgment of whether such sounds are indeed functionally adequate, cannot be based entirely on instrumental analyses, but rather must appeal to the judgments of mature language users who can listen to infant sounds and identify them as meeting requirements for phonetic sound classes. Any instrumental analysis procedure designed to categorize speech-like sounds in terms of functionally adequate units would have to mimic the perceptual activities of mature listeners. If it failed to mimic them, it would fail in its task of determining the functional potentials of the sounds. Thus, if we wish to judge the speech potential of sounds produced by infants, we must use real listeners to provide standards of recognition.

The problem with using real listeners is, of course,
that not all real listeners will hear the same message when
presented with the same signal. In fact the same listener
may not hear the same message on different occasions. A
variety of illusions, individual differences, and language
background differences clearly influence the sounds perceived
by the human listener. Such facts impose upon the data
resulting from transcriptional studies of speech (whether
infant or adult) a subjectivity and an observation error
that need to be kept clearly in mind in the evaluation of
those data (see Bush et al., 1973; Oller and Eilers, 1975).

One aspect of a well-motivated approach to transcription
is the use of transcribers whose language biases have been
limited by training with international phonetics, and who
have been sensitized to perceptual illusions. Another safe-
guard is the use of multiple transcribers and a recording of
transcriptional disagreements. To the extent that listeners
agree consistently on the categorization of particular sound
features, evidence mounts that the sounds have functionally
significant potential. To the extent that sounds are not
heard equivalently, they are ambiguous as to functional
potential.

Instrumental analyses can be used to successfully supplement transcription and attempt to determine what features
of the acoustic signal account for the particulars of tran-
scriber judgments. In addition, of course, the acoustic
analyses can provide quantitative data on certain features
in a way that transcription cannot. For instance, in studying
the onset of voicing in stop-like elements of infant babbling
Preston, Yeni-Komshian, and Stark (1967) used acoustic
analyses in such a way that the preference of infants to
produce unaspirated stops (as described in a number of
transcriptionally-based studies) can be specified in terms
of voice-onset-time (VOT) in milliseconds. The results not
only correspond well with the transcription studies in suggesting a preference for unvoiced unaspirated plosive sounds,
but they provide a basis for understanding how the transcription judgments may have been made.

Acoustic analysis becomes an even more important tool
in the description of the vocalizations of earlier infancy,
prior to the onset of adult-like "canonical" syllables. In
early infancy, there are many sounds produced that are
neither canonical syllables nor vegetative sounds. Among
these speech-like sounds are cooing, squealing, playful

yelling, etc.(cf. Oller, 1978). During these early phases, the metaphonological descriptions necessary to show the relationship of the sounds with speech can profitably rely on instrumental analyses of timing, pitch contours, resonance patterns, etc. However, even at these earlier ages, the use of auditory based judgments of the infant utterances by trained adult listeners is important.

The kinds of transcriptions and/or categorizations that can be made of these early utterances are clearly different from those that can be made later. Because canonical syllables are either rare or absent, the use of segmental notations tends to leave false implications of adult-like timing patterns unless the system of symbols includes representations of the timing aberrations that commonly occur in early infant sounds. Further, there is a need for more emphasis on the vocal quality, the pitch contours, the segmental durations, etc. than in post-canonical analyses. In general, the reliability of the segmental judgments of pre-canonical vocalizations is lower than that of post-canonical sounds. Still, the judgments of adult listeners about the speechiness of the infant sounds are needed if we are to address the goal of assessing the extent to which infant sounds could function as speech.

Relatedness of early infant sounds and speech.

Just as analogies can be drawn between late babbling and meaningful speech, relationships between early vocalization (precanonical sounds) and speech can be determined. Oller (1980) offered interpretations of early vocalizations as manifestations of an emerging capacity for speech. In this view each stage of vocal activity represents the incorporation of features of the universal phonetic code into the child's vocal repertoire. In the first months (one and two) infants often produce sounds called quasi-resonant nuclei, sounds that represent an early usage of normal phonation, but without the resonances of vowel sounds in mature speech. The phonation pattern is called "normal" precisely because it occurs as the standard phonation type in all languages. It does not occur in the infant's crying or other less speech-like sounds.

In the next two months (three and four), infants commonly produce cooing sounds. These sounds involve articulation of the dorsum of the tongue (and perhaps the epiglottis) with the palate. Because the sounds involve articulation, they

represent the incorporation of this crucial speech feature
into the infant's sound system. All languages involve the
articulation of vocal structures during the production of
normal phonation. However, the cooing sounds differ from
speech in that they do not commonly involve fully resonant
vowel-like elements and do not normally involve syllabic
timing patterns.

During the next few months (five-seven) the infant
commonly produces a wide variety of sounds, each type suggestive of an important metaphonological development: 1) fully
resonant sounds (vowel-like productions) representing the
incorporation of resonance as a contrastive parameter, 2)
squealing and growling, representing an exploration of the
ends of the pitch and vocal quality dimensions exploited by
languages, 3) yelling, representing an exploration of the
amplitude dimension, 4) raspberries (labial trills and
vibrants), representing the development of lip articulation,
and 5) marginal babbling, a vocal type in which articulation
and fully resonant nuclei are combined in proto-syllables
that only lack the proper timing relationship of consonant
and vowel as it occurs in mature spoken languages.

The canonical stage usually begins in the eighth or ninth
month of life. Infants then produce babbling combining vowel-
like and consonant-like elements with proper timing (CV transitions without breaks and not longer than 120 ms). The most
salient instances of early canonical utterances are in reduplicated babbling (including sounds that might be transcribed
as [papapa...], [tatata...], [mamama...], etc. Parents commonly note that their infants suddenly sound like they are
talking when reduplicated babbling begins. From the perspective of the development of a speech capacity, with the
beginning of canonical babbling the infant has incorporated
the timing patterns of syllables in natural languages.

One needn't assume that the infant is actively involved
in the process of developing a speech capacity (though Oller,
1981, has suggested infants may be so involved) in order to
conclude from the above analysis that even in the early stages
of infant sound production, there is a relationship between
infant vocalizations and speech. It is not certain that the
infant is trying to develop a speech capacity, and it it not
certain the infant needs to practice the commonly occurring
pre-canonical and babbling sounds in order to develop a speech
capacity, but it is clear that the emerging capacity for
speech shows itself in the vocalizations of this period. The

appearance of crucial metaphonological features of phonetic codes is systematic and shows month-by-month progress toward a broad capacity to employ and combine in complex sequences a variety of features of adult-like phonetics. By the end of the first year of life, the pre-meaningfully speaking infant is already producing a variety of phonetic shapes that are neatly suited and ready to function as words. And indeed, "mama", "papa", "tata", etc. tend to be among the nursery repertoire of real words for children in a wide variety of cultures.

Similarities of babbling cross-culturally

The fact that there tends to be a cross-cultural inventory of nursery words (cf. Ferguson, 1964) is suggestive (given the relationship of babbling and early speech) of the idea that babbling should be similar across differing linguistic environments. Indeed, of sounds produced by babies in the canonical stage, the cross-cultural similarities are striking. Existing infant data cut across a wide variety of language environments: Japanese (Nakazima, 1962), Norwegian (Vanvik, 1971), Arabic (Preston et al., 1967), French (de Boysson-Bardies et al., 1980), English (Cruttenden, 1970) and many others. All the studies report the common usage of canonical syllable types from a limited inventory. The syllables include (in IPA transcription) [pa, ta, ma, na, wa, ja] and occasionally a few others. Interestingly, the syllables included in this short list are virtually universal syllable types in mature spoken languages.

Although it is clear that there are similarities of syllable types produced by infants from widely different language backgrounds, it does not necessarily follow that there are no discernible differences attributable to early linguistic experience. The search for such differences, if they exist, however, is an empirical matter, and thus far, for infants in the first year of life, the search has not shown conclusive evidences of differences. The widely cited belief of Weir (1966) (based on pilot work) with tape-recorded babbling of a Chinese and an American infant, misled many to think that the search had already succeeded. After her death, a group of her students completed the study of adult discrimination of cross-cultural babbling (including proper controls to insure experimental blindness of observers) and found listeners were unable to identify the language background of babbling babies (Atkinson, McWhinney, and Stoel, 1970). Olney and Scholnick (1976) later

attempted a similar study and found no discrimination of
Chinese and American babies' babbling. Eady (1980) in instrumental study of pitch parameters in babbling of Chinese
and English-learning infants, failed to find reliable differences. Since the Chinese and English languages use pitch
features quite differently, and because pitch is a highly
salient feature of speech, one might have expected a high
probability of success in finding differences between these
infant language groups.

Recent work in our own laboratories (Oller and Eilers,
in press) has focused on the segmental sounds of canonical
babbling in English and Spanish-learning infants. Spanish
and English were chosen because they are quite different
kinds of languages in the segmental phonetic realm and might
yield especially clear evidence of specific language experience effects on babbling. Employing a framework similar to
the one used to illustrate the relationship of babbling and
speech within a single language (Oller et al., 1975), the
proportions of various speech sound classes occurring in the
two infant linguistic groups were compared. The results of
the study are summarized in Figure 10-1. Each data point
represents a ratio of one sound type to another (specified
on the abscissa) for either seven Spanish or seven English-
learning infants. Each ratio provides an independent comparison of the two language groups in their production of
segmental features of speech. Notice that the lines con-
necting these ratios follow each other closely, and that, in
no case do the differences between the English and Spanish
data points exceed a single standard deviation (as displayed)
from the mean ratios. Not only do the data show no significant differences between the babbling of the two groups, but
they also illustrate and quantify the extensive similarity of
babbling in the two.

It was reasoned that the failure to find audible differences between the pronunciations of Spanish and English-
learning infants in a transcriptional study might be a result
of inability of listeners to note subtle differences. Possibly
an acoustic analysis of some feature on which the two languages differed substantially might show differences in the
infant productions. In keeping with this reasoning, in a
subsequent study, Eilers, Oller, and Benito-Garcia (1981)
examined the same data corpus for possible differences
between the two groups in the production of stop consonant-
like elements. The feature of voice onset time (one on which
English and Spanish are notably different) was investigated

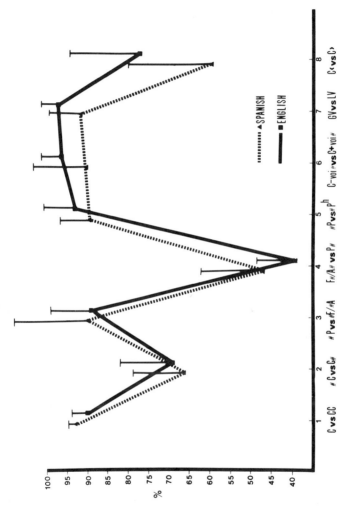

Figure 10-1. Ratios of Sound Types for Spanish-Learning and English-Learning Infants

231

using instrumental acoustic analysis. Even with the relativel
large data corpus available in the study, it was not possible
to discern differences in the two groups in their usage of
the feature of voice onset time.

What these studies show is that the attempt to find
cross-linguistic babbling differences will be difficult at
best. Even if differences do exist, they may be overwhelmed
by similarities in any empirical study. To find differences
will require a level of fine tuning of our approaches that
has as yet not been achieved.

The future of infant vocalization research

The achievements of the past in the study of infant
speech-like sound production have offered us certain undeni-
able conclusions: 1) there is extraordinary similarity of
sound types produced in late canonical babbling and in
speech; 2) early vocalizations of the pre-canonical period
manifest the emergence of a capacity for commanding many
crucial metaphonological features; and 3) there are striking
similarities of babbling in infants from widely different
language groups. The work has not, however, addressed a
variety of ultimately important issues: 1) what is the role
of specific linguistic experience in the sounds of babbling?
Are there differences between babbling in different linguistic
environments? 2) what is the role of auditory experience
independent of specific linguistic content in the appearance
of pre-canonical infant speech-like sounds? Do deaf infants
produce pre-canonical speech-like sounds which are different
from normal infants? 3) is it necessary for infants to
babble in order to prepare the speech capacity, or is the
phenomenon merely a reflection of the capacity's emergence?
4) is it possible to use the form of infant babbling as an
effective diagnostic indicator of ultimate communicative
disorders?

To address the unanswered questions, we have some of the
necessary framework tools. We know that both transcriptional
and instrumental analysis procedures will be valuable and
we have substantial knowledge of how to approach comparative
studies using both metaphonological and concrete phonological
theory to provide standards of comparison. It is clear that,
at this time, a concerted empirical effort describing vocalizations of babies from a wide variety of languages and handi-
capping conditions can be fruitful in beginning to answer
the questions above. But the progress we have made in the

past 10 years has been as much theoretical as empirical, and it seems reasonable to expect that in the next 10 years the answers we will find will depend as much on the appearance of new ways of looking at the questions as on the stolid development of a broader data base. Toward the time when further progress in the understanding of the development of the capacity for speech can be reported, we can look forward with the awareness that the understanding of normal communication development is one of the keys to the understanding of mature linguistic abilities, and is further a key in the establishment of more useful approaches to remediation of phonological disorders.

Acknowledgment

This paper is based on research supported by the Mailman Foundation and by NIMH Grant MH 30634.

REFERENCES

Atkinson, K.B., McWhinney, B. and Stoel, C. "An experiment in the recognition of babbling" Papers and Reports on Child Language Development, Number 1, Stanford, 1970.

de Boysson Bardies, B., Sagart, L. and Bacri, N. "Phonetic analysis of late babbling: A case study of a French child" Journal of Child Language 8:511-524, 1981.

Bush, C.N., Edwards, M.L., Luckau, J.M., Stoel, C.M., Macken, M.A. and Peterson, J.D. "On specifying a system for transcribing consonants in Child Language" Child Language Project, Committee on Linguistics, Stanford University, 1973.

Cruttenden, A. "A Phonetic Study of Babbling" British Journal of Dis. of Communication Vol. 5, No. 2:110-118, October, 1970.

Eady, S. "The onset of language-specific patterning in infant vocalization" Master's Thesis, Department of Linguistics, University of Ottawa, 1980.

Eilers, R.E., Oller, D.K. and Benito-Garcia, C.R. "The acquisition of voicing contrasts in Spanish and English-learning infants and children: A longitudinal study" Paper presented at the Acoustical Society of America Convention, Miami Beach, 1981.

Ferguson, C.A. "Baby talk in six languages" American Anthropology 66:103-114, 1964.

Jakobson, R. Kindersprache, Aphasie und Allgemeine Lautgesetze (Uppsala: Almqvist and Wiksell), 1941.

Lewis, M.M. Infant Speech: A Study of the Beginnings of
Language (New York: Harcourt, Brace and World), 1936.

Lynip, A.W. "The use of magnetic devices in the collection
and analysis of the preverbal utterances of an infant"
Genetic Psychology Monographs 44:221-62, 1951.

Menyuk, P. "The role of distinctive features in children's
acquisition of phonology" Journal of Speech and
Hearing Research 11:138-46, 1968.

Murai, J. "The sounds of infants: their phonemicization and
symbolization" Studia Phonologica 3:17-34, 1963.

Nakazima, S.A. "A comparative study of the speech developments of Japanese and American English in childhood"
Studia Phonologica II:27-46, 1962.

Oller, D.K. "Infant vocalizations and the development of
speech" Allied Health and Behavioral Sciences 1:523-549,
1978.

Oller, D.K. "The emergence of the sounds of speech in
infancy" in Yeni-Komshian, G., Ferguson, C. and Kavanagh, J. (eds.) Child Phonology, (New York: Academic
Press), 1980.

Oller, D.K. "Infant vocalizations: Exploration and reflex-
ivity" in Stark, R.E. (ed.) Language Behavior in
Infancy and Early Childhood (Elsevier: North Holland
Publishing Co.,), 1981.

Oller, D.K. and Eilers, R.E. "Phonetic expectation and
transcription validity" Phonetica 31:288-304, 1975.

Oller, D.K. and Eilers, R.E. "Similarities of babbling in
spanish and english-learning babies" Journal of Child
Language, (In Press).

Oller, D.K., Wieman, L.A., Doyle, W. and Ross, C. "Infant
babbling and speech" Journal of Child Language 3:1-11,
1975.

Olney, R.L. and Scholnick, E.K. "Adult judgments of age and
     linguistic differences in infant vocalization" Journal
     of Child Language 3:145-156, 1976.

Preston, M.S., Yeni-Komshian, G. and Stark, R.E. "Voicing in
     initial stop consonants produced by children in the pre-
     linguistic period from different language communities"
     Johns Hopkins University School of Medicine, Annual
     Report of Neurocommunications Lab., No. 2:305-323, 1967.

Vanvik, Arne. "The phonetic-phonemic development of a Nor-
     wegian child" Norsk Tidsskrift for Sprogvidenskap
     XXIV, Oslo, 1971.

Weir, R.H. "Some questions on the child's learning of phon-
     ology" in Smith, F. and Miller, G. (eds.) The Genesis
     of Language, (Cambridge, Mass: M.I.T. Press), 1966.

DEVELOPMENT OF PSYCHOLINGUISTIC BEHAVIOR:
THE EMERGING INFLUENCE OF COGNITIVE THEORY

Roberta L. Klatzky
University of California, Santa Barbara

The title of this text, "The Development of Psycholinguistic Behavior," raises an immediate question. Just what
is "psycholinguistic behavior"? More specifically, what is
the impact of that prefix, "psycho"? Why not just "linguistic
behavior"? What is there about children's language and its
development that is a psychological, and not simply a linguistic, phenomenon?

The answer to these questions today is very different
from what it might have been a couple of decades ago when
the field of psycholinguistics was in its infancy. The contributions of psychology to the study of language development
have changed dramatically over this period, so much so that I
think the historical perspective is invaluable to the understanding of developmental psycholinguistics as it was conducted in the "Chomskian" era, and then as it seems to be
evolving today. This chapter straddles two related issues:
What psycholinguistic phenomena can be observed in children's
development and how our view of these phenomena has changed
over the years.

To begin, I address the question of what psycholinguistics is in general. Linguistics is often defined as the
study of language. According to an admittedly narrow definition, linguistics studies language as a logical system, not
as a human behavior. In this sense, the study of computer
language, dolphin language, bird song, or whatever, could be
considered a linguistic endeavor. Psycholinguistics is, in
contrast, the study of language as a component of the human
cognitive system, and as it is manifested in human behavior.
To psycholinguists, the internal structures that represent
linguistic knowledge, the internal processes that operate on
this knowledge, and the external behaviors that express this
knowledge, are all embedded in the broader psychological
domain.

237

Actually, linguistics has evolved as something other than what my initial definition implies; that is, as more than the study of language in the abstract, or even <u>human language</u> as an abstraction. Many aspects of linguistic theorizing are psychological theorizing as well. The intuitions of humans (generally, of linguists!) have long been used to deduce what knowledge is held by speakers of a language. Chomsky called this knowledge linguistic "competence." He proposed further that the human brain held at least some linguistic competence from the time of birth. Clearly, his was a psychological theory, not a purely linguistic one. Linguists have talked not only about language per se, but about language as communication -- again, invoking psychological considerations.

The fact that both psychologists and linguists have been interested in language as a human communicative competency somewhat obscures the differences between them. In looking at developmental psycholinguistics, in particular, it becomes difficult to determine where linguistics stops and psychology begins. However, by taking the historical view, we can define this boundary more clearly. From the historical perspective, it is apparent that the relative contributions of linguistics and psychology to the study of language development have been dynamic rather than stable. A clear trend is for developmental psycholinguistics to become ever more psychological, so that the ratio of "psycho" to "linguistics" (at least, linguistics as defined by my initial statement) has decidedly increased with time.

Early developmental psycholinguistics

With these introductory remarks in mind, let us briefly review developmental psycholinguistics in the era immediately following Chomsky's (1957, 1965) classic papers on grammar. During this time, the study of child language was clearly under the Chomskian influence. A principal goal was to characterize children's language as a formal structure; essentially a linguistic, not a psychological intention. It is interesting to note what was happening in adult psycholinguistics at that time. A large number of studies was conducted to verify (or potentially disconfirm) that there existed, in the human mind, counterparts of the theoretical constructs of Chomskian theory. For example, given the importance of transformational rules in the grammar, experiments were conducted to explore the effects of the transformational complexity of sentences on comprehension and memory (e.g.,

Miller and McKean, 1964). Other studies addressed whether Chomsky's deep-structure/surface-structure distinction was relevant to human behavior (e.g., Blumenthal, 1967). As the final outcome of these efforts, Chomsky appears to have fared only moderately well as a psychologist. His major failing in this regard was an overemphasis on syntactic structures at the expense of semantics and pragmatics. But, notwithstanding flaws in his grammar as a psychological theory, its impact on students of language development was profound.

The goal of developmental psycholinguistics became to devise grammars for children's speech output that were comparable to Chomskian descriptions of adult speech. It was thought that these grammars should show successive approximations to the adult model. An outstanding example of this work is the pivot/open grammar devised for children's one and two-word utterances (Braine, 1963; McNeill, 1966). Although various forms of this grammar were developed, a simple version is as follows: Two classes of words are isolated, a small class of "pivots" and a larger class of "open words." Their possible combinations are described by phrase-structure rules, which generate "sentences" consisting of open words alone, open words in sequence, or a pivot plus an open.

Children's acquisition of transformational rules also came under scrutiny. The development of question-asking and negation were traced through stages of successive approximation to adult syntax (Klima and Bellugi, 1966). In the earliest stages (in rough temporal correspondence with the stage described by the pivot/open grammar), the syntactic devices were minimal: Questions were simple statements produced with a rising tone or prefaced by a question word such as what. Negative sentences were simply affirmatives preceded or followed by a negative term such as no. Gradually, the surface devices by which these speech acts were accomplished became complex. Auxiliary verbs were added and became the loci for tense markers. Word order was modified in accordance with the need to invert subject and verb in questions. The negative term moved into its position inside the sentence. Children's grammars were, in short, looking more adult.

There is much to be gained from the syntactic approach, but it has turned out to provide a rather incomplete account of what children are learning about language. Developmental psycholinguists soon began to reveal two distinct kinds of problems (reviewed by Brown, 1973). One concerned flaws in

the syntactic descriptions per se. This arose particularly
in the pivot/open descriptions for one and two-word utterances.
These grammars were found not to apply to all children, and
even those children who used pivots appeared to do so under
constraints that were not captured in the grammar's simple
rules. (For example, some theoretically grammatical construc-
tions were, in practice, avoided.) The second type of problem
with the syntactic grammars is more fundamental. It is that
in providing only syntactic descriptions, these theories fail
to capture the rich semantic basis for children's speech.
Developmental psycholinguists, as a result, have turned away
from the syntactic approach, placing their emphasis on richer
descriptions. This movement is part of a larger trend toward
exploring the cognitive underpinnings of language in tandem
with language itself. This symbiotic relationship between
cognition and language forms the subject matter of the "new"
developmental psycholinguistics, to which I now turn.

Later trends in child language

     As I said earlier, today's developmental psycholinguistics
appears to be far more psychological in its orientation than
previously. I will describe three general research areas
that illustrate this trend. The first is the development of
rich, semantically based, "grammars" for children's early
utterances, which essentially replace the earlier pivot/
open approach. The second research area is directly concerned
with semantic development; it investigates the acquisition of
meanings for single words. The third research area is one
that is discussed more extensively in the chapter by Carol
Prutting, so I allude to it only briefly. It represents an
extreme in the cognitive approach to language development, in
that it looks at linguistic competence without a direct manifestation in language. I refer to work on language as communication, which examines such phenomena as the communicative
skills which precede overt use of language and the relationship between language and the extralinguistic context.

     Let us first take another look at grammars for children's
one- and two-word utterances. In the early 1970s, Lois Bloom
(1970) and Roger Brown (1973) developed descriptions for these
utterances that were richer than the pivot/open accounts then
prevalent. The new descriptions went beyond the surface form
of what was uttered to the child's underlying semantic intent,
which was inferred from the context of the utterance as well
as the words themselves. Brown suggested that the "pivot
look" of children's speech at the two-word stage was an

artifact of the child's intention to indicate certain semantic
relations. Those relations, such as pointing out recurrence
by using the word "more," were expressed by a small set of
terms. Because these terms were used over and over with
various content words, the resulting utterances produced a
"pivot look." Even more important in these theories was the
decomposition of utterances that had previously been classified as two "open" words, according to the semantic roles
played by those two words. Brown claimed that most of these
utterances portrayed a relatively small set of semantic
roles, such as the agent of an action plus the action, or an
action plus acted-upon-object. This semantically based
description is more directly related to Fillmore's (1968)
case grammar than to Chomsky's.

Brown has characterized the semantic roles of two-word
utterances as the culmination of Piaget's (1937) sensory-motor
stage of intelligence. This theorizing again reflects the
contemporary interest in relating language acquisition to
cognitive development in general. During the sensory-motor
period, the child learns that objects endure in time and
space, and he or she begins to understand causal relations.
The two-word utterances of early speech seem to capture these
understandings. Early sentences serve such functions as
naming and noting the recurrence of objects and identifying
the initiators of actions. As Brown put it (1973, p. 199),
"Where should the meanings of the first linguistic construc-
tions come from if not from the sensorimotor intelligence
which directly precedes them?"

The second research area that I shall use to illustrate
later trends in developmental psycholinguistics is semantics
of the single word, that is, the study of how children develop
word meanings. At the outset, we can conceive of two views
of this phenomenon. One is that the development of word
meanings is simply a matter of learning what labels apply to
known concepts. In this view, children's learning of words
begins with their having fully developed, well differentiated,
adult-like, conceptual categories. Their task, then, is
simply to learn the labels for the categories. The child
might still make errors along the way. For example, seeing a
dog and cat together and hearing the label "cat," the child
might misidentify the word's referent and call the dog a cat.
Another source of errors might arise when a child has no label
for a category. Lacking the label "cat," the child might
choose to apply the label "dog," knowing full well that cats
are not dogs, but not having a better word for cats. There

is some evidence that children make some errors on just this
basis. For example, children may make more errors in overt
naming than in comprehension tasks, suggesting the concept is
known but the name can't be generated (Thomson and Chapman,
1977).

Another view of semantic development is that it is virtually indistinguishable from the development of concepts in
general. That is, the proper use of word labels develops in
tandem with cognitive knowledge about their referents. In
this view, children's errors -- such as applying a category
name too broadly or too narrowly -- derive from ill-formed
concepts, rather than from misapplication of labels for well-
formed concepts. There is evidence to support this view as
well as the first.

Probably, both theories of semantic development are true
to some extent. Children may misapply names for concepts
they understand fully, and in other cases, they may have to
learn the concept and label together, misapplying the label
because they don't understand the adult form of the concept.
The latter case is particularly interesting in the context
of this talk, because it ties mastery of words to the mastery
of concepts, and thus it nicely illustrates the cognitive
approach to developmental psycholinguistics. Eve Clark (e.g.,
1973) has expressed this view as a specific model of semantic
development. It holds that children develop conceptual categories feature by feature. When a concept has too few
features, the use of the name for that concept may be too
broad. For example, if the concept of dogs includes only
such features as four-legged, furry, and domesticated, it
will not suffice to differentiate dogs from cats. A single
label may then be applied to both.

As a final illustration of newer trends in developmental
psycholinguistics, I turn to certain language-related phenomena that are not, strictly speaking, linguistic at all. I
include here two distinct topics. One is contextual influences on linguistic behavior. The other is prelinguistic
communicative behavior. I am discussing these topics together because they illustrate a common trend, which is to treat
children's language development as part of a more general
growth in communicative skills. When we talk about children
as communicators, rather than mere speakers, we must look
not only at the content of speech, but its function. This
leads us very naturally to look at the context in which
speech occurs, and also to nonlinguistic means of performing
similar functions.

Since this topic is taken up in depth in Carol Prutting's chapter, my comments are brief. In fact, I mean simply to point out the interest in prelinguistic communicative skills, and to let Prutting take up that discussion in earnest. About the related topic of language-in-context, I have a bit more to say.

I have already given brief mention to the topic of speech in context. You may recall that I characterized the early descriptions of children's one- and two-word utterances as linguistic, and the later descriptions as psychological. An essential difference between these two types of descriptions is in the reliance on context. One needs context to determine the underlying semantic roles played by words in one- and two-word utterances. Looking at their context is what made the richer, semantic descriptions of these utterances possible.

Context has also been important in studying the acquisition of meanings for single words -- namely, deictic terms. Deictic words (from deixis, the Greek for "pointing") are those that acquire meaning in part from the context of their utterance. They include pronouns like I and you, demonstrative adjectives like these and that, and locatives like here and there. One needs to understand the place and person of the speaker, in contrast to an addressee, in order to understand the meanings of these words. Their meaning will also shift with the semantic content of the conversation. For example, "here" can mean either at UCSB or on this spot, depending on the discussion.

Recently, Leda Tfouni and I conducted a study of deictic acquisition. We explored several factors which should affect children's mastery of deictic words. One factor we manipulated was whether the child was an active participant in discourse or a spectator to the discourse of others. We asked children to act out commands using the words this, that, here, and there, such as, "Put this elephant on the white square," or "The fence goes over there." We reasoned that since appropriate use of deictic words varies with the identity of the speaker, children's comprehension would suffer if that identity were made more difficult to monitor. In particular, comprehension would be impaired if children were spectators to discourse, in which case they would have to monitor two potential speakers other than themselves, in comparison to the situation where children were active participants, in which case they could identify the speaker directly as either

"self" or "other." The prediction that performance with the
deictic words would be worse in the spectator condition was
confirmed. This same effect was absent when errors on nondeictic words were considered (e.g., color identification
errors), as would be expected, since speaker identity is not
integral to the meaning of the nondeictic words.

Interestingly, in this same study, children's difficulties with deictic terms were dramatically reduced if the
words were accompanied by pointing gestures. Deictic word
use has been viewed as the culmination of a process that
begins with children's pointing (Bates, 1976; Clark, 1978).
That is, the communicative function served by deictic words
in adult discourse is assumed to be accomplished by the preverbal child through pointing. Our results indicate that even
when children have mastered deictic words, locative motor
acts such as pointing may be a residual component of their
meanings, so that the overt use of a pointing gesture along
with a word can aid in the word's comprehension. In contrast,
pointing had no effect on children's errors with nondeictic
words in this task.

Summary and Prognostication

To briefly summarize this talk, I have given several
examples of contemporary research topics in child language.
These included studies of the form and semantics of children's
first utterances and the development of word meanings. I have
emphasized in this discussion that the study of children's
language is being undertaken hand in hand with the study of
children's cognitive development. Thus, for example, two-
word utterances are seen as expressing sensory-motor competence. The use of single words is seen as reflecting the
growth in conceptual knowledge. And when we turn to single
words that express deictic concepts, semantics is seen as
inseparable from the ability to communicate, which begins
even before children manifest language.

I have contrasted this approach to linguistic behavior
with a prior approach, which I called more linguistic than
psycholinguistic. The earlier, linguistic approach arose
under heavy influence from Chomskian theory. The new approach
combines both linguistic theory and cognitive-developmental
theory.

Where are we heading? I predict that the marriage
between cognition and developmental psycholinguistics will

be a lasting one. Psycholinguistic theory will be increasingly influenced not only by theories of cognitive development, but of adult cognition. There may be a potential danger here, if we should end up relegating studies of language development to a secondary status, so that they are directed solely by cognitive theories. It will be important to consider as well those aspects of language development that are unique to language. But there will be strong gains from the cognitive influence on developmental psycholinguistics. Cognitive psychology is a rapidly advancing discipline. It straddles broad areas; yet it can make concrete assumptions at the microprocess level. Its predictions are tested by the rigors of data collection and statistical evaluation. The theories of cognitive psychology promise to be a powerful heuristic for the study of psycholinguistic development.

REFERENCES

Bates, E. Language and Context: The Acquisition of Pragmatics (New York: Academic Press), 1976.

Bloom, L.M. Language Development: Form and Function in Emerging Grammars (Cambridge, Mass.: MIT Press), 1970.

Blumenthal, A.L. "Prompted recall of sentences" Journal of Verbal Learning and Verbal Behavior 6:203-206, 1967.

Braine, M.D.S. "The ontogeny of English phrase structure: the first phase" Language 39:1-13, 1963.

Brown, R.W. A First Language: The Early Stages (Cambridge, Mass.: Harvard University Press), 1973.

Chomsky, N. Syntactic structures (The Hague: Mouton), 1957.

Chomsky, N. Aspects of the Theory of Syntax (Cambridge,Mass.: MIT Press), 1965.

Clark, E.V. "What's in a word? On the child's acquisition of semantics in his first language" in Moore, T.E. (ed.) Cognitive Development and the Acquisition of Language (New York: Academic Press), 1973.

Clark, E.V. "From gesture to word: on the natural history of deixis in language acquisition" in Bruner, J.S. and Garton, A. (eds.) Human Growth and Development: Wolfson

College Lectures, 1976 (Oxford: Oxford University Press),
1978.

Fillmore, C.J. "The case for case" in Bach, E. and Harms,
R.T. (eds.), Universals in Linguistic Theory (New York:
Holt, Rinehart & Winston), 1968.

Klima, E.S. and Bellugi, U. "Syntactic regularities in the
speech of children" in Lyons, J. and Wales, R.J. (eds.)
Psycholinguistics Papers (Edinburgh: Edinburgh University
Press), 1966.

McNeill, D. "Developmental psycholinguistics" in Smith, F.
and Miller, G.A. (eds.) The Genesis of Language (Cambridge, Mass.: MIT Press), 1966.

Miller, G.A. and McKean, K.E. "A chronometric study of some
relations between sentences" Quarterly Journal of
Experimental Psychology, 16:297-308, 1964.

Piaget, J. The Construction of Reality in the Child, first
edition, 1937 (New York: Basic Books), 1954.

Thomson, J.R. and Chapman, R.S. "Who is 'Daddy' revisited:
the status of two year olds' over-extended words in use
and comprehension" Journal of Child Language 4:359-
375, 1977.

DEVELOPMENT OF COMMUNICATIVE BEHAVIOR

Carol A. Prutting
University of California, Santa Barbara

My main interest has been to look at the psycholinguistic
and sociolinguistic literature and to apply these insights
to my own field of speech/language pathology. I have primarily dealt with the language of schoolage children as well
as adults, but with the shift that has occurred in pragmatics,
a different theoretical paradigm has led me into being more
interested in infants. Klatzky, in the previous chapter,
reviewed quite a bit of the Chomsky influence, and I'd like to
go over a few issues that may make this chapter clearer.

Chomsky wrote his major book in 1957 which started a
linguistic revolution. This book was a departure from Harris'
structural linguistics. Nineteen years later, Bates (1976)
came out with some very important ideas about looking at
language in context, and I mark that as the beginning (almost
two decades later) of another theoretical shift in the fields
of psycholinguistics and sociolinguistics. The differences
have been talked about in terms of a formalist theory with a
syntactic emphasis and a functionalist paradigm with an
emphasis on pragmatics. One way to describe the shift
is about the differences in definitions for each paradigm
(Bates and MacWhinney, in press). To Chomsky language consists of a set of sentences: that is how language was defined.
Under a functionalist paradigm, Bates would define language
as an instrument for social interaction, which is quite a
different way of looking at language. In terms of its function, formalists describe language as the expression of
thought; whereas, to a functionalist, language is a means to
communicate. Competence, of course, has meant very different
kinds of things for both camps. The formalists believed
competence was the ability to produce, comprehend, and judge
grammaticalness. That greatly influenced the field of
research application to speech and language pathology which
has really concentrated on syntax. This level was central to
the entire language system. For the functionalists, competence lies in the relational system and that system needs
to be viewed within a relationship and then it had to do with

social competence; it is rooted in social interaction, and
some have said it is a complex commitment to social interaction. That is what language is about. In terms of a hier-
archial framework, the formalists view syntax as central to
their viewpoint, and then semantics in order of importance,
and then pragmatics, although most of the formalists did not
address that issue. For them context was the internal aspect
of the sentence, and anything outside of the sentence was not
always looked at in the way it needs to be looked at at this
point. For the functionalist, the pragmatic level is central
to the understanding of the communicative system, and that is
the prime focus and the framework from which to look at
semantics and syntax. The hierarchies of importance run
from pragmatics to semantics to syntax, just the opposite
of the formalist focus. The emphasis, of course, for the
Chomsky era was the acquisition and use of linguistic rules.
The emphasis today is on pragmatic rules which include both
linguistic and non-linguistic rules.

Bates and MacWhinney (in press) described these two
theories: one is an "inside" theory, which is the formalists'
point of view focusing on innate explanations for language
acquisition; and the new paradigm shift, the pragmatic aspect
on language in context, is more of what they calls an "outside"
theory which involves the social and cognitive reasons for
acquisition. Another interesting difference is that Chomsky's
theory was a contemporary theory. You could read about him
in Time magazine. We all know about this contemporary theory.
People have a hard time understanding pragmatics and what to
do with it in relationship to linguistics. I think one of the
reasons stems from the fact that its origin comes from
American Pragmatism which was dealt with about 1887 by the
famous philosopher Charles Pierce and then by Austin, Searle,
and Wittgenstein, who utilized that notion with regard to
language. Pragmatics comes directly from the area of philosophy, and our prior two decades of research utilized a linguistic framework. I think that makes a difference. People
are not as familiar, it is not a contemporary theory. The
notions about pragmatics span over a century. The generali-
ties from the 60s and 70s stated that all children pass
through the same stages of language acquisition. That was
one generality that most people believed. The second generality was, while they pass through the same stages, they
do so at various rates. The other emphasis was on innate
factors; and an important difference, in terms of our unit
of measurement between the formalist and the functionalist,
is that the focus was always on the individual with the

Chomsky paradigm. It was on how does the individual comprehend, produce, and judge grammaticalness. The emphasis now -
although I'm not willing to make too many generalizations
because this is a relatively new area - is what is called
the homology model - that non-linguistic behavior can be
related to linguistic behavior. In other words, the environmental factors are of great importance for acquisition in a
pragmatic paradigm. The other focus with regard to measurement is that the focus is not on the individual but on the
dyad, and I think that's one of the major contributions that
pragmatics has already made, going away from the utterance
which is an individual's behavior and going to the discourse
measurement which is dyadic type of information. In terms of
the research, Klatzky, in the previous chapter, covered the
acquisition of syntactic structure, described the pragmatic
focus and semantic relationships and so forth. One issue
of interest today is the idea of relatedness or dependency
among social, linguistic, and cognitive behaviors.

Bates (1979) has talked about four specific non-
linguistic behaviors that occur sometime, she thinks, between
9-13 months, and she has some empirical data to support this
opinion. It is predicted that these behaviors must be present
in order for symbolic acquisition or first words to develop.
According to Bates, the behaviors are: imitation, symbolic
play, tool use (both non-social tool use where you use an
object to get something and social tool use where you use a
person to do something you cannot do, such as wind up a toy),
and the last prerequisite (according to Bates) is communicative intention. Of course all of this is done without the
first word. Showing, pointing, and giving behavior are real
indicators of later symbolic development. It is a very
interesting proposal because what it means is that we have
a much richer ability to diagnose early communicative
behaviors at the first year level. Bates' prediction is
that if you find that these behaviors are not present or up
to threshold then you would expect some type of deficit.
Of course, language disordered children are interesting to
look at in view of Bates' beliefs. At present we are
exploring the acquisition of tool years in Down's Syndrome
children because they are easily identified at a very early
age. We are attempting to see if Bates' theory holds up.
Either way we stand to learn a great deal more about children
with disordered language. That is one whole area of pragmatic research which I think is very exciting. I am always
reminded of Bever's (1975) beautiful example in terms of a
search for causal factors. He talks about his hypothesis

regarding how kangaroos hop. He states that kangaroos generally hop by using both legs and tail. If, however, one
observes hopping-impaired kangaroos, whether due to infant
childhood disease or genetic mutation that damaged the legs
and tail, what we would undoubtedly find is that such kangaroos manage to rely relatively more on whatever organs
remain intact, leading to aberrant hopping but hopping nevertheless. Whatever the clinically observed results, as we
said earlier, we would know a little more than before about
the organization of hopping in a normal kangaroo. It is
tricky to find dependence or to ask dependency-related questions across sub-systems like linguistic, social, and cognitive. This is one of the major interests at this point in
child language.

A second area for pragmatics has to do with the functions
of language. Functions or intentions grow out of the speech
act theory that Austin (1962) and Searle (1969) at one time
discussed. Lately child language investigators are not as
interested in the overt form of an utterance as they are in
the function. In other words, "How does language serve an
individual?" is one of the questions that is being asked. In
child language literature it's "How does language serve the
needs of the child?" Interestingly enough, Halliday (1975)
and Dore (1974) as well as others are looking at these phenomena in acquisition. Piaget asked that question back in 1926
when he looked at peer interactions. He was always way ahead
of his contemporaries.

Conversational rules are a third area of research. Just
as we are interested in how the child adds the gerund ending,
and when they do this, and when they put in the auxiliary
verb, we are now interested in asking when a child learns
to turn-take verbally, non-verbally, and so forth. When
does a child learn to manipulate a topic, change topic,
terminate topic, etc.? We are interested in conversational
rules that are considered verbal rules as well as non-verbal
rules such as physical proximity. When does a child learn
how far to stand from a speaker and a listener? In our
society, as in every society, these conversational rules can
be documented. For instance with regard to physical proximity
in our society it is 18-24 inches; if you go to England and
measure proximity it may be different. The non-linguistic
rules lend themselves to the same empirical type measurements
as the linguistic rules, and we have in the past neglected the
nonverbal components of communication.

Stylistic variations are the fourth area. Examples from Kuhl's chapter in terms of "motherese" have to do with stylistic variations. People are now interested in asking how do caretakers change their speech to youngsters, and older children, and so forth. Now they're interested in asking, "How do language disordered children and normal children talk to peers, talk to people of higher status, talk to older people?" There is much research interest in that area. I think basically the departure has been to go away from the sentence and to expand the context in which communication can be studied. To my way of thinking, that's a very important contribution. We looked very much at those two-word utterances and longer utterances, but it was always the individual's overt linguistic behavior that we were trying to analyze.

Now you can see, the four areas under pragmatics have to do with prerequisites to symbolic acquisition which may be housed in the paralinguistic and non-verbal behavior of the child during the first year. In addition, we are looking at functions or how does language serve the child? Can the child ask for an object and regulate someone else's behavior? We are asking about the child's conversational rules. How does the child manage the flow of discourse? This ability is as important as putting an auxiliary verb in a sentence, and it is outside of the sentence. The last area is stylistic variations. How does a child learn that it's alright to say this to a peer but not to grandmother? These are all of the social awareness type of knowledge.

One thing I've noticed in my particular field is that we seem to move on a continuum from a very narrowly described context which we feel comfortable with and then we (over the years) venture out and expand upon the context from which we can study phenomena. We have certainly crawled out of the sentence and it is getting very scary because now to study communication is to study the world or to study what it means to be human. There is not anything that is not communication, and that is what people in the pragmatic area are finding. When you put a paper over your head and sleep on the Long Island Railroad, you are communicating to the fellow next to you. I think we will see a retreat basically back to less of a context in which we will study communication, but right now it is wide open. We can just about do anything and make it a pragmatic study. I'm talking about Speech-Language Pathology, and child language from my point of view was very influenced by Bates. Nobody invented it.

Another aspect that I think is important for me to talk
a little bit about is in terms of Bever's (1975) comment. I
think the important questions are to look at social, cognitive, linguistic, and non-linguistic behavior in relationship
to each other. There are some very nice data, for instance,
about non-linguistic behavior as a regulator for linguistic
behavior. For example, when children are placed in a triad
situation, they will use eye gaze and physical proximity and
postural shifts, all non-linguistic, to regulate verbal turn
taking. We need to use a multi-channel analysis and right
now we are primarily focusing on verbal behavior. To look at
those four areas in relationship to each other I think will
be very important.

Some of Curtiss' work at U.C.L.A. suggests that you can
find severely disordered children who, for instance, have
very high linguistic structures and cognitively are very low
and the opposite phenomena as well (personal communication,
1981). I'm not sure what we'll find, but it seems to me we
need to add to the cognitive-linguistic analysis and social
analysis and start looking at social development because
that seems to be important. Then, in addition, instead of
microanalysis, as researchers do, I think we need to get into
a macro-analysis. I'm trying to do social validation studies
using a macro-analysis. I'm interested in asking questions
like: given that there's a different style of interaction,
can you change this clinically? If you do change this, is
it facilitative in any way or linguistic in social development? According to a recent paper by Nelson (1981), the
type of interaction dictates not only the functional content
of language but what parts will be learned first and how
those parts will be put together or broken down for reassembly.
She is giving a great deal of credit to the interaction. The
particular kind of interaction will dictate not only the
function and content of the language but which parts are
learned first. The question I'm interested in asking is not
so much do styles of interaction change and differ, of course
they do, but what difference does that make? We're not sure
how we'll proceed in terms of that research. Clinically I'm
interested in asking something about changing patterns that
are basically tied to personality. I have several examples
of a child exhibiting social tool use; for instance, the
investigator would wind up a little toy and the child doesn't
have the motor control to do that, and then the child wanted
to do it but couldn't. One example of social tool use would
be to take the wind up toy and hand it to the adult. Look at
the adult. We have several behavioral phenomena we're looking

at now -- gaze, some type of motor response, and so forth.
Now we're looking at Down's Syndrome and normal infants in
relationship to tool use, and trying to work out how to do
observational research with 10-month-old infants, and it is
very difficult.

This next type is the social validation work that I'm
interested in. This study involved a Down's Syndrome adole-
scent and a normal person who was just taken off the street
and asked if he would come in and talk for about 20 minutes.
Observing the linguistic and pragmatic behavior of the boy
with Down's Syndrome, one can see that he's very unintelligible at times and has a very concrete vocabulary, but prag-
matically he was very good in terms of his social behavior.
Who would be the better communicator? That client has a linguistic problem and a second client we would judge clinically
as having a pragmatic problem: lack of initiation, lack of eye
contact, hands in pockets, unattentive posture, etc. What
I've been trying to do is show tapes holding the normal communicative partner constant and asking people in classrooms
to make judgments about these communicators. The question
I'm asking basically is, what is more penalizing: a linguistic
problem (phonological, syntactic, or semantic) or a pragmatic
problem (either linguistic or non-linguistic)? I guess the
reason I asked the question, as most researchers do, I think
I know the answer. The pragmatic problem would be much more
penalizing. And that is how all of the data seem to be
going. In other words, there's an interesting thing that has
happened. We've spent two decades of having speech and
language professionals correct phonology, syntax, and semantics. Now, all of a sudden, pragmatics has come about and we
must turn our attention to children and adults who have just
a pragmatic problem. There doesn't seem to be a cognitive
linguistic one. They're talking about it as being a personality problem, and this is not our role. A pragmatic problem
or a social one are the same. We use pragmatics in the field
of language, all language problems are really social in terms
of the effects the behavior has on other people.

Can one really define abnormal on a pragmatic scale?
Do we know that range of normal pragmatic behavior? How do
you judge someone's personality? What is personality but
one's non-verbal, paralinguistic, and verbal behavior! One's
communicative abilities mirror what others think about that
person. My guess is that personality is disclosed by the
manner in which you communicate and people read you by your
communicative behaviors.

We should be interested in how disordered people regulate
their relationships with others through communication because
communication is really a vehicle (defined in a pragmatic
paradigm at least) which allows one to initiate, maintain,
and terminate relationships. To me it is a very nice movement to incorporate with phonology, syntax, and semantics.
We've been around for about 57 years and we're coming full
circle. Van Riper (1939) defined a speech disorder as one
which calls attention to itself, interferes with communication, or causes a person to be maladjusted. Today we define
a language and speech disorder outside of a relationship
often and in reference to a test score. And so to me it is
a healthy swing, but it is not a new idea. When I went to
school we spent three weeks on how to establish rapport; that
was important. Many curricula don't have any type of counseling courses, but are very well schooled in the internal
structure of the sentence. We need to bring the disorder
back to the person -- I think the pragmatic shift will help
us do this.

REFERENCES

Austin, J. How to do Things with Words (Cambridge: Harvard
    University Press), 1962.

Bates, E. Language in Context (New York: Academic Press),
    1976.

Bates, E., Benigni, L., Bretherton, I., Camaioni, L. and
    Volterra, V. The Emergence of Symbols (New York:
    Academic Press), 1979.

Bates, E. and MacWhinney, E. "Functionalist approaches to
    grammar" in Gleitman, L. and Wanner, E. (eds.) Language
    Acquisition: The State of the Art (New York: Cambridge
    University Press), in press.

Bever, T. "Some theoretical and empirical issues that arise
    if we insist on distinguishing language and thought"
    Annals of New York Academy of Science 76-83, 1975.

Chomsky, N. Syntactic Structures (The Hague: Mouton), 1957.

Curtiss, S. Linguistics Department, University of California,
    Los Angeles, personal communication, 1981.

Dore, J. "A pragmatic description of early language development" Journal of Psycholinguistic Research 4:343-350,
1974.

Halliday, M. Learning How to Mean (London: Edward Arnold),
1975.

Klatzky, R. "Development of psycholinguistic behavior: the
emerging influence of cognitive theory," in Gerber, S.E.
and Mencher, G.T. (eds.) The Development of Auditory
Behavior (New York: Grune & Stratton, Inc.), this
volume.

Kuhl, P.K., "The perception of speech in early infancy: four
phenomena" in Gerber, S.E. and Mencher, G.T. (eds.) The
Development of Auditory Behavior (New York: Grune &
Stratton, Inc.), this volume.

Nelson, C. "Individual differences in language development:
implications for development and language" Developmental
Psychology 17:170-187, 1981.

Piaget, J. The Language and Thought of the Child (London:
Routledge and Kegan Paul Ltd), 1926.

Pierce, D. "How to Make Ideas Clear" Popular Science Monthly
12:286-302, 1978.

Searle, J. Speech Acts: An Essay in the Philosophy of
Language (New York: Cambridge University Press), 1969.

Van Riper, C. Speech Correction: Principles and Methods
(Englewood Cliffs, New Jersey: Prentice Hall), 1939.

Wittgenstein, L. Philosophical Investigations (New York:
Macmillan Publishing Co.), 1958.

Part IV

Conclusions

THE DEVELOPMENT OF AUDITORY BEHAVIOR:
IMPLICATIONS FOR HABILITATION OF HEARING IMPAIRED CHILDREN

Agnes H. Ling Phillips
Montreal Oral School for the Deaf, Montreal, Quebec

Over the course of two tightly packed days, a great deal
of information on early auditory behavior was presented. In
this paper, however, I will restrict myself to a consideration
of some of the more important implications which might be
drawn from Conference contributions, from the perspective
of a habilitationist and educator of hearing impaired children
whose special concern is to help hearing impaired children
acquire spoken language. This is most easily achieved
through the maximal use of residual hearing, a goal which
in turn is facilitated by early identification of hearing
loss and provision of a family oriented habilitation program.
The more we can learn about the development of auditory
behavior, the better we will be able to diagnose hearing loss
in infancy and devise programs which will permit us to
develop each child's auditory potential.

Development of Auditory Potential

Recent advances in the knowledge of anatomical development of the auditory system were described by Hunter-Duvar
and by Ruben (this volume). The quality of auditory stimulation experienced by the developing auditory system can bring
about anatomical, physiological and behavioral changes. In
the absence of auditory stimulation, the auditory centers of
the brain do not develop. For clinicians and educators working
with hearing impaired children, this finding is of major
importance. Hearing loss should be identified as soon as
possible after birth, the infant should be fitted with appropriate amplification and provided with the widest possible
range of meaningful auditory experiences.

The effective use of residual hearing is of relatively
recent origin. Although one can find mention of auditory
training for deaf children as far back as the 18th century
(see Wedenberg, 1951 for a review), it has only been with the

advent of high quality individual hearing aids that the
residual hearing capacities of hearing impaired children
could be exploited to the full (Ling, 1975).

Although vision has generally been considered the most
important sense modality for hearing impaired people, a number
of professionals have viewed audition as a primary avenue for
learning language, even for children with very limited hearing
(Huizing, 1951; Wedenberg, 1954; Whetnall, 1955; Ling, 1959;
Pollack, 1964; Griffiths, 1967; Beebe, 1975).

The rationale for the use of an auditory approach was
based partly on successful experience and partly on reports
of the drastic effects of sensory (visual) deprivation on
newborn animals (Scott & Marston, 1950; Wiesel & Hubel, 1965;
Riesen, 1966). Furthermore, evidence from studies of children
who had been brain damaged in early versus late childhood,
contributed to the notion of a critical period for language
development (Lenneberg, 1967).

The question of a critical, or at least optimal period,
for language learning is of considerable importance in
relation to the provision of intervention programs for hearing impaired infants and their parents. Kyle (1978) has
criticized the concept of a critical period, and Bench (1978)
has further questioned the value of intervention from birth.
However, in view of the findings of Hunter-Duvar (this volume)
and also of Ruben & Rapin (1980) physicians, audiologists,
and educators should once again be sensitized to the crucial
importance of identifying hearing loss in infancy and immediate implementation of a comprehensive program of auditory
management. So that valuable time is not lost when hearing
status is in doubt, or when a hearing aid has not been fitted
or for some reason is not available, parents should be encouraged to stimulate their child's hearing by talking
directly into the ear, a technique used by Wedenberg (1951)
and earlier proponents of an auditory approach.

Early Identification of Hearing Loss

This current focus of identification is on the screening
of infants deemed to be at high risk of being hearing impaired (Mencher, this volume). Mass screening of neonates
using behavioral techniques was initiated by Downs & Sterritt
(1964), and also undertaken by others (e.g., Ling, Ling &
Jacobson, 1968; Feinmesser & Tell, 1971; Mencher, 1974).
Problems encountered in such early screening programs (Ling,

Ling & Doehring, 1970) led to a search for stimuli which would
more readily elicit reliable and valid responses (e.g. Eisenberg, 1971; Ling 1972; and Gerber, this volume); to the development of instrumentation which would obviate the need for
observers (Simmons & Russ, 1974; also Hecox, Mendel, this
volume); to propel researchers into in-depth studies of the
auditory capacities of both newborn and older babies (Eisenberg, 1976; Kuhl, Trehub, this volume); and to a restriction
of the target population to those infants considered to be at
high risk of having a hearing impairment (Mencher, this
volume).

While the importance of testing high risk infants is not
questioned, over reliance on this strategy may lead to the
late diagnosis of children who do not fall into one of the
at risk categories (e.g., children whose hearing impairment
is recessive genetic in origin). This implies the need for
additional procedures. Of crucial importance is the alerting
of physicians to the serious consequences of childhood hearing
impairment, to its many causes, and to important indicators
that hearing might not be intact. Doctors also neeed to be
brought up to date about recent advances in audiological
assessment (e.g. Hecox, Mendel, Gerber, Wilson, this volume).

Assessment of Infant Auditory Capacities

The contribution of several conference participants
(viz. Hecox, Mendel, Gerber, Wilson, Kuhl, and Trehub) taken
together indicate that it is possible to obtain an impressive
amount of information about the auditory capacities of infants
through the use of ever more sophisticated techniques. From
all accounts, it appears that the auditory system is highly
developed at birth, and further that by twelve months of age
certain responses (e.g., auditory brain stem responses, Hecox,
this volume) are comparable to those obtained with adults.
Wilson (this volume) went so far as to challenge the notion
of "development." While much remains to be done, the pains-
taking research so far undertaken with normal hearing subjects should allow for more detailed and accurate assessment
of children with impaired hearing and the selection of appropriate amplification for infants. As Mencher (this volume)
pointed out, clinical practice generally lags a year or two
behind research. Interaction between clinical audiologists
and researchers studying the auditory perceptual capacities
of infants should be encouraged. Comparative studies of
normal hearing and hearing impaired infants may also contribute to the acceptance, rejection, or refinement of theoretical models of auditory perception such as that suggested

by Doehring (this volume). Of importance would be the study
of the effects of auditory training and experience in developing residual hearing.

Habilitation of Hearing Impaired Infants

   The presentations by Oller, Klatzky and Prutting have
implications for certain aspects of early intervention.

   Oller (this volume) discussed in some detail the vocal
repertoire of infants from about six months of age, stressing
the universal and non-random character of the syllable
sequences used. The implication for those working with
hearing impaired babies is to develop those same babble
patterns, since they are presumably important precursors of
fluent speech (see D. Ling, 1976; A.H. Ling, 1977). Such
syllabic babble can be elicited from hearing impaired babies,
but as with normal hearing infants, it occurs subsequent to
a period of several months during which a repertoire of vowel
sounds is acquired in the context of vocal play (Lach, Ling,
Ling, & Ship, 1971). Progress depends to a large extent on
what the infant is able to hear of the vocalizations of others
and how he can relate them to his own productions. Parents
will therefore need help to ensure that their hearing impaired
infants quickly adjust to full time use of their hearing
aids (Ling & Ling, 1978).

   Pragmatic aspects of linguistic development were discussed during the Conference by both Klatzky and Prutting.
In her overview of the field of psycholinguistics, Klatzky
commented that initial focus was on how syntax emerged in the
young child. Subsequently, research turned towards the
semantic aspects of language, and most recently, pragmatics
has held center field. Prutting further elaborated on the
current role of pragmatics in the study of communicative
development. Apparently the young normal hearing child
becomes increasingly sensitive to the context in which interaction takes place, and learns to modify the form and content
of his utterances accordingly. Such skill is often lacking
in the hearing impaired person. This may be because educators
of the hearing impaired have generally placed greatest emphasis on the development of syntax (e.g. Fitzgerald, 1949;
Russell, Quigley & Power, 1976; Blackwell et al., 1978). While
it will long continue to be necessary to find more effective
means of developing adequate use of syntactic structures
among hearing impaired children, attention must also be given
to ensuring that a wide range of semantic notions are acquired,

and that communicative skill in a broad range of situations is mastered.

The emergence of psycholinguistics as a field of study had a significant impact on the reappearance of sign language as a medium of instruction for hearing impaired children. It was hoped that the use of sign language during infancy, in conjunction with the use of hearing aids, speech-reading and speech teaching, would ensure the optimal means of development. Appealing as the concept of total communication is, it is extremely hard to put into effect. A major consequence has been a de-emphasis on the role of hearing and the development of spoken language. In practical terms, it is very difficult for the educator to ensure optimal conditions for the various component parts of total communication. The focus has been on developing communication first by means of sign language and then later working on auditory training and speech. In view of confirmation that a lack of auditory stimulation and experience is likely to lead to permanent damage to the auditory centers of the brain (Hunter-Duvar, this volume), more careful attention will have to be given to ensuring that all hearing impaired children have optimal opportunity to make use of whatever little hearing capacity they possess. This is especially so if there is to be any serious attempt to develop speech. While the results of earlier studies (e.g., Montgomery, 1966) showed that the speech of children using sign language was no worse than that of children in oral classes, careful reading of the research shows that the speech was generally unintelligible. More recent research indicates that maximum use of residual hearing from infancy, coupled with a systematic approach to speech teaching can result in highly intelligible speech at least for some profoundly hearing impaired children (Ling & Milne, 1981).

Skeptics (e.g., Moores, 1978) have questioned the benefits of early intervention. Certainly the mere discovery of hearing loss in infancy in no way guarantees markedly higher standards of literacy or speech intelligibility. Although the effects of a severe or profound loss may be mitigated, they are not negated by its early discovery. Audiologists and educators of the hearing impaired may have been overly optimistic about the benefits of early amplification and have underestimated the need for comprehensive management which includes parent counselling (Luterman, 1979; Moses & Van Hecke-Wulatin, 1981), guidance relating to techniques which will facilitate acceptance of hearing aids, and a carefully devised program concerning the development of auditory, vocal, linguistic and communication skills within the context of the baby's cognitive, social and emotional needs and his place in the family.

Conclusion

No radically new solutions to habilitation appeared to emerge from the Conference, but rather confirmation of earlier findings and refinements of techniques which should permit more efficient detection and diagnosis of hearing impairment. Implications for habilitation indicate the need for increased emphasis on the earliest possible development of auditory perceptual capacities. Perhaps the most important outcome of the Conference for me was an increased awareness of the enormous potential to be gained by a sharing of knowledge among researchers working in related areas, and among researchers, clinicians and educators working with hearing impaired children. On the one hand, clinicians and educators need to become increasingly skilled at evaluating the results of research, and to become enthusiastic partners in joint research projects. On the other hand, researchers need to listen to and respect the viewpoints of clinicians and educators who are engaged in diagnostic and habilitative work on a daily basis.

ACKNOWLEDGEMENTS

I wish to thank Donald G. Doehring, Ph.D. for helpful editorial comments.

REFERENCES

Beebe, H. "Deaf children can learn to hear" Talk, 75:6-8, 1975.

Bench, J. "The basics of infant hearing screening: why early diagnosis?" in Gerber, S.E. and Mencher, G.T. (eds.), Early Diagnosis of Hearing Loss (New York: Grune & Stratton), 1978.

Blackwell, P., Engen, E., Fischgrund, J.E. and Zarcadoolas, C. Sentences and Other Systems: A Language and Learning Curriculum for Hearing-Impaired Children (Washington, D.C.: A.G. Bell Assoc.), 1978.

Downs, M.P. and Sterritt, G.M.   "Identification audiometry
    for neonates: a preliminary report"   Journal of Auditory
    Research   4:69-80, 1964.

Eisenberg, R.B.   "Pediatric audiology: shadow or substance?"
    Journal of Auditory Research   11:148-153, 1971.

Eisenberg, R.B.   Auditory Competence in Early Life: The Roots
    of Communicative Behavior   (Baltimore, MD: University
    Park Press), 1976.

Feinmesser, M. and Tell, L.   "Progress Report: evaluation of
    methods of detecting hearing impairment in infancy and
    early childhood" (V.S.P.H.S. - M.C.H.S. Project 06-48D-Z)
    Department of Otolaryngology, Hadassah Hospital, Jeru-
    salem, Israel, 1971.

Fitzgerald, E.   Straight Language for the Deaf   (Washington,
    D.C.: The Volta Bureau), 1949.

Griffiths, C.   "Auditory training in the first year of life"
    in Proceedings of the International Conference on Oral
    Education of the Deaf, Vol. 1, (Washington, D.C.: A.G.
    Bell Assoc.), 1967.

Huizing, H.   "Auditory training"   Acta Otolaryngologica
    Supplement   100:158-163, 1951.

Kyle, J.G.   "The study of auditory deprivation from birth"
    British Journal of Audiology   12:37-39, 1978.

Lach, R., Ling, D., Ling, A.H. and Ship, N.   "Early speech
    development in deaf infants"   American Annals of the
    Deaf   115:522-526, 1970.

Lenneberg, E.H.   Biological Foundations of Language   (New York:
    John Wiley & Sons, Inc.), 1967.

Ling, A.H.   Schedules of Development in Audition, Speech,
    Language, Communication for Hearing Impaired Infants &
    their Parents   (Washington, D.C.: A.G. Be-l Assoc.),
    1977.

Ling, D.   "The education and general background of children
    with defective hearing in the borough of Reading"   Un-
    published research associateship thesis, Cambridge
    University Institute of Education, England, 1959.

Ling, D. "Response validity in auditory tests of newborn infants" _Laryngoscope_ 82:376-380, 1972.

Ling, D. "Recent developments affecting the education of hearing-impaired children" _Public Health Reviews._ 4:117-152, 1975.

Ling, D. _Speech and the Hearing Impaired Child: Theory & Practice._ (Washington, D.C.: A.G. Bell Assoc.), 1976.

Ling, D. & Ling, A.H. _Aural Habilitation: The Foundation of Verbal Learning in Hearing-Impaired Children_ (Washington, D.C.: A.G. Bell Assoc.), 1978.

Ling, D., Ling, A.H. & Doehring, D.G. "Stimulus response and observer variables in auditory screening of newborn infants" _Journal of Speech and Hearing Research_, 13:9-18, 1970.

Ling, D., Ling, A.H. and Jacobson, C. "Detection and treatment of deafness in early infancy" _Canadian Family Physician_ 14:47-52, 1968.

Ling, D. and Milne, M.F. "The development of speech in hearing-impaired children" in Bess, F.H., Freeman, B.A. & Sinclair, J.S. (eds.) _Amplification in Education_ (Washington, D.C.: A.G. Bell Assoc.), 1981.

Luterman, D. _Counseling Parents of Hearing-Impaired Children_ (Boston, Mass.: Little, Brown & Co.), 1979.

Mencher, G.T. "A program for neonatal hearing screening" _Audiology_ 13:9-18, 1974.

Montgomery, G.W. "The relationship of oral skills to manual communication in profoundly deaf adolescents" _American Annals of the Deaf_ 111:557-565, 1966.

Moores, D.F. _Educating the Deaf_ (Boston, Mass.: Houghton, Mifflin Co.), 1978.

Moses, K.L. & Van Hecke-Wulatin, M. "The socio-emotional impact of infant deafness: a counselling model" in Mencher, G.T. & Gerber, S.E. (eds.) _Early Management of Hearing Loss_ (New York: Grune & Stratton), 1981.

Pollack, D. "Acoupedics: a uni-sensory approach to auditory training" Volta Review 66:400-409, 1964.

Riesen, A.H. "Sensory deprivation" Progress in Physiological Psychology 1:117-147, 1966.

Ruben, R.J. and Rapin, I. Plasticity of the developing auditory system. Annals of Otology, Rhinology and Laryngology 89: (4, pt. I), 303-311, 1980.

Russell, W.K., Quigley, S.P and Power, D.J. Linguistics and Deaf Children (Washington, D.C.: A.G. Bell Assoc.), 1976.

Scott, J.P. and Marston, M.V. "Critical periods affecting the development of normal and maladjustive social behavior in puppies" Journal of Genetic Psychology 77: 25-60, 1950.

Simmons, F.B. and Russ, F.N. "Automated newborn hearing screening, the Crib-o-gram" Archives of Otolaryngology 101:1-7, 1974.

Wedenberg, E. "Auditory training of deaf and hard of hearing children" Acta Otolaryngologica Suplement 94, 1951.

Wedenberg, E. "Auditory training of deaf and hard of hearing children" Acta Otolaryngologica Suplement 110, 1954.

Whetnall, E. "The deaf child" Practitioner 174:375-384, 1955.

Wiesel, T.N. and Hubel, D.H. "Extent of recovery from the effects of visual deprivation in kittens" Journal of Neurophysiology 28:1060-1972, 1965.

Theoretical Aspects of Auditory
Perceptual Development

Donald G. Doehring
McGill University, Montreal, Quebec

During the past ten years there has been increasing
interest in studying the auditory perceptual abilities of infants (Eimas and Miller, 1981; Yeni-Komshian, Kavanagh, and
Ferguson, 1980). This impressive body of new research was
stimulated by findings which seemed to indicate that speech
sounds are processed by a unique form of perception called
categorical perception (Liberman, Cooper, Shankweiler, and
Studdert-Kennedy, 1967), and that infants may be born with
the ability to perceive speech sounds categorically (Eimas,
Siqueland, Jusczyk, and Vigorito, 1971), perhaps by means of
special linguistic feature detectors (Eimas and Miller, 1978).
The discovery of innate speech perception mechanisms would
have been a major breakthrough in psychological research, and
would have supported the views of linguists regarding the in-
nateness of language abilities (cf. Chomsky, 1965). However,
there are now several different kinds of evidence against the
special nature of speech perception. Nonspeech sounds as well
as speech sounds are perceived in a categorical manner (Cutting
and Rosner, 1974); animals as well as humans perceive speech
in a categorical manner (Kuhl and Miller, 1978); and there may
not be specialized linguistic features, or even, perhaps, any
auditory feature detectors at all (Remez, 1979; Remez, Rubin,
Pisoni, and Carrell, 1981). Proponents of the view that
speech perception is unique and at least partially innate
have modified their explanations in the face of this evidence
(cf. Eimas, Tarttar, and Miller, 1981; Studdert-Kennedy,
1980).

Fortunately, the negative findings regarding innate
speech perception abilities have not restored the study of
infant auditory perception to its former state of neglect.
The invaluable legacies of this stimulating but unsuccessful
theoretical venture are the objective methods for evaluating
infant auditory perception that had been adapted from methods
for studying infant visual perception (Eimas et al., 1971) and

269

from methods for the audiological evaluation of infants
(Wilson, this volume). With these new methods, investigators
have continued their efforts to determine the number of different speech sounds that infants can discriminate (see
Eilers, 1980; Jusczyk, 1981; and Trehub, Bull, and Schneider,
1981a for recent reviews), have begun to study the extent to
which infants categorically perceive nonspeech sounds
(Jusczyk, Rosner, Cutting, Foard, and Smith, 1977), and have
also begun to explore the auditory analogue of visual perceptual constancy (Kuhl, 1980). This new and exciting field
of research is dominated by a concern with methodology, and
rightly so. Infants have a very limited but rapidly-evolving
response repertoire, and the utmost care is needed to devise
methods that will yield valid inferences for as wide a range
of ages as possible (Trehub, Bull, and Schneider, 1981a).

Further details of ongoing research in infant auditory
perception were given in other chapters. In the present
paper, I discuss some of the theoretical considerations
that can help to guide this research. Even though methodological concerns are presently at the forefront, another
theoretical framework is needed to replace the special theory
of speech perception. We are still faced with the problem
of accounting for the manner in which the infant comes to
attach meaning to specific patterns of sound waves. If we
espouse interactive theories (cf. McClelland and Rumelhart,
1981), it might not be possible to explain infant auditory
perception without explicitly indicating how meaning is
attached to auditory input. I begin by discussing theories
of how the infant might perceive non-meaningful sounds,
and then speculate briefly about the role of meaning. The
purpose of this discussion is to suggest that even a very
skeletal and provisional theoretical framework can be of help
in indicating potentially fruitful directions of research on
the development of infant auditory perception.

Psychoacoustics and Discrimination

Psychoacoustics arose from the efforts of early psycho-
physicists to construct scales of psychological pitch and
loudness discrimination along the measurable acoustic dimensions of frequency and intensity. Early investigators
succeeded in mapping the ability of mature listeners to discriminate changes in the frequency and intensity of pure tone
within the audible range (Licklider, 1951). These abilities
seem relatively invariant, which might suggest that they are

universal and innate. It would seem logical to postulate that
they are either available at birth or shortly after birth as
a function of the maturation of the auditory system. Can we
assume that these psychophysical discrimination abilities provide the basis for auditory perceptual learning? If so, we
might have an answer to the question posed by Gibson and
Gibson (1955) as to whether perceptual learning involves differentiation or enrichment, at least with respect to auditory
perception. Although traditional psychoacoustics did not
really provide a theory, it is worthwhile to determine
whether infants can resolve changes in acoustic parameters
with the same precision as adult listeners. Research of this
type has been initiated by Trehub and her colleagues (Schneider,
Trehub, and Bull, 1979; Trehub, Bull, and Schneider, 1981a).

An argument for the application of traditional psychoacoustic concepts to the study of infant auditory perception
is that the current infant research paradigms are very much
like those of traditional psychophysics. New paradigms might
be sought among traditional psychophysical methods (Guilford,
1954). An argument against the use of traditional psychoacoustic concepts is that infants do not normally listen to
discrete pure tones of varying intensity in the presence or
absence of white noise, but to a conglomeration of different
complex sounds, often dominated by the nearby vocalizations
of caretaking adults and the sounds of their own respiration
and vocalization. Modern psychoacoustic research has studied
the discrimination of complex acoustic stimuli by adults
(Pastore, 1981). It might be useful to study such abilities
in infants to determine whether they are as invariant and
universal as abilities to discriminate pure tones. The extension of traditional and modern psychoacoustics to the study
of infants lies largely in the future and will require a great
deal of methodological ingenuity. The extent to which such
research seems worthwhile depends on one's implicit or explicit
theory of auditory perceptual development.

Discrimination and Categorization

Traditional psychoacoustics is concerned with the precision with which the listener can resolve changes in acoustic
parameters (Robinson and Watson, 1972). The ability to discriminate small changes in sounds has adaptive significance
in the jungle, in traffic, and in conversations. Of equal
importance is the ability to perceive different sounds as
equivalent, even when they vary considerably as a function of

distance, reverberation, source, and immediate acoustic context. Rapid and automatic decisions regarding equivalence are
needed for adaptive responses to animal cries, automobile
engines, and spoken language. I will use the term categorization to describe such responses.

Theoretical interest in categorization arose in the early
stages of modern cognitive psychology (Bruner, Goodnow, and
Austin, 1956), not from traditional psychophysics, but the
categorical perception paradigm (Liberman et al., 1967) can be
considered a tool of psychoacoustics to the extent that
acoustic parameters and stimulus-response contingencies are
precisely controlled. Early work on categorical perception
suggested that discrimination is very poor within categories
and only becomes precise at the boundary between categories
(Liberman et al., 1967). Such a phenomenon would be of great
theoretical significance, since it could suggest either the
evolutionary development of innate regions of non-
discrimination for adaptive purposes, or the perceptual
unlearning of innate distinctions within adaptively-significant
categories. Research on infant auditory perception might
appear to support the former theory (Eimas et al., 1971;
Jusczyk et al., 1977), but there is now some question as to
whether the poor discrimination within categories is an artifact of the memory requirements of the categorical perception
task (Aslin and Pisoni, 1980). Infants and adults may be
able to discriminate and categorize at the same time. From a
theoretical point of view, it is not difficult to postulate
two separate levels of processing, either of which might be
attenuated or accentuated for adaptive purposes.

Although the status of categorical perception is un-
certain at present, it is important to determine the infant's
relative abilities for making coarse categorizations and fine
discriminations. Research design might be facilitated by more
consistent definition of the constructs of discrimination and
categorization within a single theoretical framework. At
present there is some ambiguity in the distinction between
discrimination and categorization in research on infant auditory perception, since the most common type of study assesses
the infant's ability to discriminate phonological categories.
To the extent that the two categorical stimuli (e.g., the
speech sounds /ba/ and /pa/) and the acoustical context
remain acoustically unchanged, we can say that discrimination
is being studied; but to the extent that there are variations
within the phonological categories or in the acoustical context from trial to trial, categorization is being studied.

This distinction can be clarified by specifying three types of categorization. The simplest type, and the one which relates most directly to discrimination, is a categorical response to a series of changes in an acoustic continuum such as rise time, voice onset time, or the direction of a formant transition, e.g., the listener classifies stimuli on one side of the phoneme boundary as belonging to Category A, and stimuli on the other side as belonging to Category B. A more complex type is what Bruner, Goodnow, and Austin (1956) called conjunctive categorization, where there is a categorical response to the attribute which defines the category, such as the phoneme /a/, despite trial-to-trial variation of irrelevant characteristics such as the speaker and the adjacent phonemes. The most complex form of categorization is what Bruner, Goodnow, and Austin called disjunctive categorization, where the defining attributes are not invariant, but may change from trial to trial as a function of whatever other attributes are present. An example of this type of categorization would be the category of voiced sounds, the defining attributes of which may vary as a function of the acoustic context (Lisker, 1978). All three types of categorization could be classified as perceptual constancy (Kuhl, 1980), since the listener makes the same response to a variety of stimuli. The degree to which discrimination and the three different types of categorization are innate may vary considerably among the four types of ability, and may also vary as a function of the types of speech sounds that are involved (Blumstein, 1980; Haggard, 1977). It is important to make clear distinctions among the four types of ability in formulating a theoretical framework that combines psychoacoustics and cognitive psychology.

Integration and Differentiation

The rather modest types of theoretical construct that define discrimination and the three types of categorization seem necessary to explain how the infant may adapt to auditory stimuli by detecting some differences and ignoring others. However, these constructs are not sufficient to explain how a given sound pattern may be perceived in a unitary manner, and how different sound patterns are perceived by the listener as separate. Is the infant born with the ability to integrate the acoustic energy from a single sound source and to differentiate the acoustic energy from different sound sources? Relatively recent theories of Jones (1976) and Bregman (1981) suggest that the integration and differentiation of sounds occurs as a function of the relative ratios of frequency,

intensity, and time within the complex acoustic signal. Sounds
that have the proper ratios with respect to the three dimensions tend to be perceived within a unitary pattern or stream,
and sounds that differ sufficiently along one or more dimensions are perceived as not belonging to the same pattern or
stream. Natural speech and nonspeech sounds are characterized
by optimal ratios among the acoustic dimensions. Sounds that
differ sufficiently, such as a buzz, a hiss, and a click
cannot be perceived in an integrated manner (Warren, Obusek,
Farmer, and Warren, 1969).

In order to perceive speech and music, it is not only
necessary to spatially integrate the simultaneously-occurring
components such as fundamental, formants, and plosive bursts,
but to integrate the temporal sequence of sounds. For effective adaptation, then, the listener must not only be able to
discriminate and categorize sounds, but to integrate the
spectral and temporal acoustic patterns of natural sounds.
The extent to which this type of ability is innate or acquired
is of obvious importance in studying infant auditory perception

The opposite side of the coin is differentiation, where
the listener must sometimes be able to perceive different
sound patterns as separate even when they are quite similar,
such as different voices in a crowd and different musical
instruments in an orchestra. Once again, optimal ratios of
frequency, intensity, and time are needed for unitary perception of a particular sound pattern in the presence of similar
sound patterns. An infant may be able to perceive an isolated
pattern of speech or nonspeech sounds in a unitary manner,
but not to differentiate that pattern from similar patterns
with the same proficiency as a mature listener. Recent
research by Trehub, Bull, and Schneider (1981b) suggests that
this may be the case. To explore such questions further,
one could adapt the types of stimuli devised by Bregman and
his colleagues (cf. Bregman, 1981) to the paradigms used with
infants.

Theoretical Model of Auditory Perception

It is undoubtedly worthwhile to separately study the
infant's ability to discriminate, categorize, integrate, and
differentiate speech and nonspeech sounds. However, such
research is most likely to be meaningful in the long run if
it is guided by a model of auditory perception, even if the
model is quite skeletal and very provisional. For illustrative purposes I have constructed a general model of auditory

perception in the mature listener, as shown in Fig. 14-1. The model is derived from the types of partially-interactive parallel processing models that have been recently proposed for reading (McClelland and Rumelhart, 1981). The model is by no means complete or final, but it does give some indication of how interactive processing might take place.

Auditory perception in the mature listener must always involve an interaction of sensory input and past knowledge. In this model, the acoustic signal results in sensory input that undergoes several stages of transformation as it is conducted through the peripheral auditory system, the auditory nerve, and the brainstem to a primary receiving area in the auditory cortex, where the transformed representation of the signal is briefly stored while preliminary analysis takes place by the extraction of acoustic cues. The percept is formed within a dynamic system designated as working memory (Baddeley, 1976; Just and Carpenter, 1980), where the products of preliminary analysis are interactively processed via a final analysis system, the details of which are shown in the lower part of Fig. 14-1. Within the final analysis system there may be interactions among the mechanisms for discrimination, categorization, integration, and discrimination. The percept is formed by interaction of the final analysis of the input with relevant past knowledge and also with current contextual information. This takes place within working memory.

Not all of the current auditory input will necessarily be processed through a single system. The listener may listen to birds through one system, speech through another system, and music through still another system. These systems may in turn be subdivided. In speech, for example, the identity, the accent, and the intonation may be processed separately from the segmental content. The systems would not, of course, be independent. This necessitates a complex model of auditory perception that defies pictorial representation at the present time.

Interactive models have their limitations. In a fully-interactive model, for example, information about temporal order might be lost. The present model, although perhaps allowing for too much interaction, is not fully interactive. There is no direct connection between brief sensory storage and stored knowledge. More important, the preliminary analysis system is the only link between brief sensory storage and the higher-level perceptual systems. One of the crucial theoretical issues pertains to the necessity for a stage of auditory analysis that always precedes higher levels of

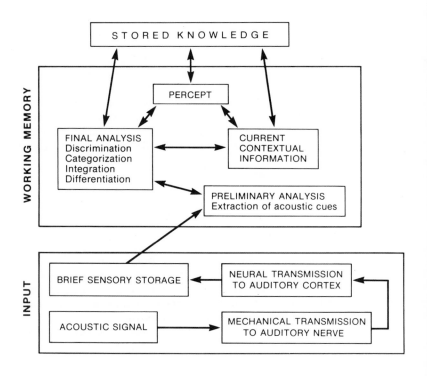

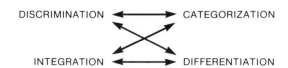

Figure 14-1. Proposed Model of Infant Auditory Perception

analysis (Pastore, 1981; Pisoni, 1981). The present model is somewhat ambiguous in this respect. Preliminary analysis provides the only link with higher stages, but it is an interactive link. The extent to which preliminary auditory analysis actually does precede further perceptual analysis is important for understanding auditory perceptual development.

Would the model shown in Fig. 14-1 be appropriate for describing the auditory perception of neonates and infants? We might expect the subcortical auditory system to be closest to maturity at birth, and stored knowledge to be least developed. The relative state of development of the intermediate parts is open to question. The developmental status of the preliminary analysis and final analysis systems is the subject of current research. Some of the mechanisms within these systems may be fully developed at birth and others may be partially developed. It seems reasonable to speculate from casual observation that by age two most children are able to discriminate, categorize, integrate, and differentiate sounds in a manner that is not noticeably deficient. We might also speculate that the neural mechanisms for brief sensory storage are fully developed or almost fully developed in the neonate, but no research has yet been carried out on this aspect of auditory perceptual development. Although brief sensory storage, which has also been designated as pre-categorical acoustic storage (Crowder and Morton, 1969), is included in almost all models of auditory perception, the process has not been as thoroughly studied as the analogous visual process (Neisser, 1967).

The course of development of the mechanisms for maintaining current contextual information in working memory, of working memory itself, and of stored knowledge are matters for speculation at this point. "Knowledge", in some sense of the term, of certain types of categories and certain types of integrated sounds may be present at birth, and tacit knowledge of the expected frequencies of occurrence and co-occurrence of particular sounds should begin to accumulate after birth, as should the types of knowledge about the associations between sounds and objects, events, feelings, ideas, and symbols that are necessary for the attachment of meaning to percepts.

Investigation of the development of the "higher" aspects of auditory perception lies in the future. Research will be influenced by changes in models of auditory perception, especially with respect to the relationship between speech and nonspeech perception. As long as we continue to define

auditory perception in terms of the interaction of sound and
knowledge, as both the earliest (Berkeley, 1709) and the most
recent (McClelland and Rumelhart, 1981) theorists have done,
the investigator of infant auditory perception must remain
aware of all components of the systems which relate sound to
knowledge.

The most difficult task for investigators of infant
auditory perception will be to determine how meaning comes
to play a role in perception, whether by simple associative
learning (an idea which is highly repugnant to many of our
colleagues in cognitive psychology and psycholinguistics) or
by some more complex process. Meaning obviously plays an
essential role in the adaptive aspects of perception. As
meaning increases, the infant should be able to respond more
rapidly and precisely to auditory stimulation. Meaning may
also qualitatively alter perception, as suggested by evidence
that infants may be superior to older children in phoneme discrimination (Barton, 1980) and perceptual constancy (Tallal,
Stark, Kallman, and Mellits, 1980). Although it is difficult
at present to incorporate meaning into working models of infant
auditory perception, this will be a challenge for future
theorists.

Models of Development

In addition to cross-sectional models which describe
auditory perception at a particular stage of development, we
need longitudinal models that describe how perception changes
from birth to maturity. Two types of model are available,
those which concentrate on infancy and those which cover the
entire period to maturity. The former type of model is of
most immediate relevance. Possible alternative models of
early development have been discussed in an excellent paper
by Aslin and Pisoni (1980). Some of these models are listed
in Table 14-1, which has been freely adapted from Aslin and
Pisoni.

Several important questions arise from consideration
of the alternative models of early development. How many of
the mechanisms involved in auditory perception are fully
developed or partially developed at birth? If not fully
used, do these abilities remain the same, or do they deteriorate? If they deteriorate, can they be reinstated by
experience? To what extent does perceptual development after
birth take the form of invariant maturational unfolding,

TABLE 14-1:   SOME POSSIBLE MODELS OF AUDITORY PERCEPTION
DEVELOPMENT (adapted from Aslin and Pisoni, 1981)

1. Fully-innate universal abilities

    a. Unaffected by experience

    b. Decay through disuse

        i. Cannot be re-established by experience

        ii. Can be re-established by experience

2. Partly-innate abilities

    a. Universal abilities that develop further by
        invariant maturational unfolding

    b. Partially-idiosyncratic abilities that are
        tuned by experience

        i. Permanent tuning

        ii. Can be re-tuned by new experiences

3. Learned abilities entirely shaped by experience

resulting in universal abilities, or follow an experientially-
guided course of special tuning? Present information about
infant auditory perception might lead us to postulate that
some of the mechanisms in the final analysis system of Fig.
14-1 are partially-developed at birth and are selectively
tuned by specific auditory experiences to which the infant
is exposed. The most peripheral aspects of the auditory
system may be most fully developed and universal, and the
central aspects may be least developed at birth and most
likely to show individual variations. The ages at which the
various abilities involved in auditory perception become fully
mature and the range of individual differences in perceptual
development must have an important bearing on the development
of spoken and written language. After we begin to understand
infant perceptual development, it may be possible to explain
further development to maturity within the context of the
hierarchical stages of cognitive development postulated by
neo-Piagetian theorists such as Fischer (1980).

Further Directions of Theory and Research

As a result of the remarkable increase in research on
infant auditory perception during the past ten years, we now
know quite a bit about the ability of infants to discriminate
between speech-sound categories (Eimas and Miller, 1981; Yeni-
Komshian, Kavanagh, and Ferguson, 1980) and are beginning to
learn more about their psychoacoustic abilities (Trehub, Bull,
and Schneider, 1981a), their abilities to categorize nonspeech
sounds (Jusczyk et al., 1977), and their abilities to make
more abstract categorizations of speech sounds (Kuhl, 1980).
Among the phenomena that remain to be investigated are the
abilities to integrate sound patterns and differentiate them
from other sound patterns. The research to date on discrimination and categorization has been made possible by the clever
adaptation of research paradigms to fit the infant's limited
response repertoire. Even more ingenuity may be needed to
devise ways of determining how well the infant can integrate
and differentiate sound patterns across spectra of frequency
and intensity and over time. As stated above, the types of
stimulus array developed by Bregman and his colleagues
(Bregman, 1981) might be appropriate for this purpose. The
high-amplitude sucking paradigm or the head-turning paradigm
might be used for studying infant integration and differentiation, or perhaps the operant procedure developed by
Friedlander (1970) might prove helpful.

It will be most interesting to find out how infant auditory perception really works. We may find that the infant is
born with auditory perceptual mechanisms that enable her to
discriminate, categorize, integrate, and differentiate sounds
with almost as much precision as the mature listener, providing we can devise research paradigms that will enable her
to demonstrate these abilities. Perhaps paradoxically, these
innate abilities would at first be used to "perceive" meaning-
less sounds, since the infant is probably not born with innate
ideas, mental images, disjunctive categories, or meaningful
associations involving linguistic and nonlinguistic sounds.

There are many other interesting phenomena that could be
studied in relation to infant auditory perception, and even
more will probably occur to us as we learn more about speech
and nonspeech perception in mature listeners. For example,
auditory perception, particularly in the infant, may not be
the type of active process described in books on Piagetian
development (cf. Flavell, 1963), where the infant becomes an
increasingly busy manipulator of objects that provide visual,

tactual, and kinesthetic stimulation. The listening infant
can lie passively in the crib and obtain auditory stimulation
without moving. He is, of course, interested enough in sounds
to actively suck in order to turn on novel but not
intrinsically-fascinating speech and nonspeech sounds in
certain experimental situations (Eimas et al., 1971). Is
auditory perceptual learning a relatively passive process
largely motivated by what we might call idle curiosity or
non-contingent pleasure in listening to such things as birds
and music? There should be ways of finding out just how much
auditory perceptual learning differs from the type of learning
postulated by theories which stress the active emission of
overt responses (cf. Gibson, 1966; Skinner, 1938). Another
important issue is the unresolved theoretical status of the
relationship between speech perception and speech production.
The developmental aspects of this complex issue are now being
considered by some investigators (Straight, 1980; Strange and
Broen, 1980).

Finally, the formulation of empirically-verified models
of auditory perceptual development should enable us to study
auditory perceptual disorders in a more effective manner.
As Rees (1981) has recently pointed out, the confusion
regarding the existence, incidence, and definition of auditory perceptual disorders (also called central auditory
disorders and auditory processing disorders) results from the
lack of a comprehensive theoretical framework. If adequate
models of auditory perceptual development can be formulated,
we may be able to determine how supposed auditory perceptual
deficits contribute to language, learning, and reading problems. Some of the auditory perceptual deficits that have been
described thus far might be explained in terms of the model
described above. The rate processing disorders described by
Tallal and her colleagues (Tallal and Stark, 1980) would
appear to be discrimination deficits, whereas difficulties
in separately perceiving simultaneously-presented syllables
on the SSW Test (Katz, 1977) could involve difficulty in
differentiating either speech sounds in particular or both
speech and nonspeech sounds. Other auditory perceptual deficits that have been listed by Rees (1981) could also be in-
terpreted with reference to the model. For example, sequencing
problems could involve difficulty at the level of integration,
as could blending and closure problems; and figure-ground
problems could involve difficulty in differentiation. Auditory
memory problems could obviously have something to do with
working memory. Expressing the characteristics of deficient
auditory perceptual processes in the terminology of a single

theoretical model should provide a useful link between basic and applied research on auditory perceptual development.

At the beginning of the last decade, many of us were convinced that speech perception was a special process that should be studied by itself. Certain cautionary voices (cf. Cole and Scott, 1974; Stevens, 1975) warned us that speech perception might not be as special as we thought, and now the theoretical tide has turned to the point where we formulate general models of auditory perception that can be applied to both speech and nonspeech perception. Whether or not the tide turns again, we are well-advised to search out the most plausible model available at any given time to guide our efforts to understand auditory perceptual development.

REFERENCES

Aslin, R.N. and Pisoni, D.B.   Some developmental processes in speech perception.   In G.H. Yeni-Komshian, J.F. Kavanagh and C.A. Ferguson (Eds.), Child Phonology. Volume 2: Perception, New York: Academic Press, 1980.

Baddeley, A.D.   The psychology of memory.   New York: Basic Books, 1976.

Barton, D.   Phonemic perception in children. In G.H. Yeni-Komshian, J.F. Kavanagh and C.A. Ferguson (Eds.), Child Phonology. Volume 2: Perception. New York: Academic Press, 1980.

Berkeley, G.   An essay toward a new theory of vision. 1709.

Blumstein, S.E.   Speech perception: An overview. In G.H. Yeni-Komshian, J.F. Kavanagh and C.A. Ferguson (Eds.), Child Phonology. Volume 2: Perception, New York: Academic Press, 1980.

Bregman, A.S.   Asking the "what for" question in auditory perception. In M. Kubovy and J.R. Pomerantz (Eds.) Perceptual Organization. Hillsdale, New Jersey: Erlbaum, 1981.

Bruner, J.S., Goodnow, J.J., and Austin, G.A.   A study of thinking. New York: Wiley, 1956.

Chomsky, N.   Aspects of the theory of syntax. Cambridge, Massachusetts: MIT Press, 1965.

Cole, R.A. and Scott, B. Toward a theory of speech perception. Psychological Review, 1974, 81, 348-374.

Crowder, R.G. and Morton, J. Precategorical acoustic storage (PAS). Perception and Psychophysics, 1969, 5, 365-373.

Cutting, J.E. and Rosner, B.S. Categories and boundaries in speech and music. Perception and Psychophysics, 1974, 16, 564-570.

Eilers, R.E. Infant speech perception: History and mystery. In G.H. Yeni-Komshian, J.F. Kavanagh and C.A. Ferguson (Eds.), Child Phonology. Volume 2: Perception, New York: Academic Press, 1980.

Eimas, P. and Miller, J. Effects of selective adaptation on the perception of speech and visual patterns: Evidence for feature detectors. In R.D. Walk and H.L. Pick (Eds.), Perception and experience, New York: Plenum, 1978.

Eimas, P.D. and Miller, J.L. (Eds.), Perspectives on the study of speech. Hillsdale, New Jersey: Erlbaum, 1981.

Eimas, P., Siqueland, E.R., Jusczyk, P., and Vigorito, D.J., Speech perception in infants, Science, 1971, 171, 303-306.

Eimas, P.D., Tartter, V.C. and Miller, J.L., Dependency relations during the processing of speech. In P.D. Eimas and J.L. Miller, (Eds.), Perspectives on the study of speech. Hillsdale, New Jersey: Erlbaum, 1981.

Fischer, K.W., A theory of cognitive development. Psychological Review, 1980, 87, 477-531.

Flavell, J.H., The developmental psychology of Jean Piaget. New York: Van Nostrand, 1963.

Friedlander, B.Z., Receptive language development in infancy. Merrill-Palmer Quarterly, 1970, 16, 7-51.

Gibson, J.J., The senses considered as perceptual systems. Boston: Houghton Mifflin, 1966.

Gibson, J.J. and Gibson, E.J., Perceptual learning-differentiation or enrichment? Psychological Review, 1955, 62, 32-41.

Guilford, J.P., Psychometric methods, Second Edition, New
    York: McGraw-Hill, 1954.

Haggard, M., Do we want a theory of speech perception? Paper
    presented at the research conference on Speech-Processing
    Aids for the Deaf, Gallaudet College, Washington, D.C.,
    23-26 May, 1977.

Jones, M.R., Time, our lost dimension: Toward a new theory of
    perception, attention, and memory. Psychological Review,
    1976, 83, 323-355.

Jusczyk, P.W., Infant speech perception: A critical appraisal.
    In Eimas, P.D. and Miller, J.L. (Eds.), Perspectives on
    the study of speech. Hillsdale, New Jersey: Erlbaum,
    1981.

Jusczyk, P.W., Rosner, B.S., Cutting, J.E., Foard, C.F., and
    Smith, L.B., Categorical perception of non-speech sounds
    by two-month old infants. Perception and Psychophysics,
    1977, 21, 50-54.

Just, M.A. and Carpenter, P.A., A theory of reading: From eye
    fixations to comprehension. Psychological Review, 1980,
    87, 329-354.

Katz, J., The staggered spondaic word test. In R.W. Keith
    (Ed.) Central auditory dysfunction. New York: Grune &
    Stratton, 1977.

Kuhl, P.K., Perceptual constancy for speech-sound categories
    in early infancy. In G.H. Yeni-Komshian, J.F. Kavanagh
    and C.A. Ferguson (Eds.), Child Phonology. Volume 2:
    Perception, New York: Academic Press, 1980.

Kuhl, P.K. and Miller, J.D., Speech perception by the chin-
    chilla: Identification functions for synthetic VOT
    stimuli. Journal of the Acoustical Society of America,
    1978, 63, 905-917.

Liberman, A.M., Cooper, F.S., Shankweiler, D.P., and Studdert-
    Kennedy, M., Perception of the speech code. Psychological
    Review, 1967, 74, 431-461.

Licklider, J.C.R., Basic correlates of the auditory stimulus.
    In S.S. Stevens (Ed.) Handbook of experimental psychology
    New York: Wiley, 1951.

Lisker, L., Rapid vs. rabid: A catalogue of acoustic features that may cue the distinction. Haskins Laboratory Status Report on Speech Research, 1978, SR-54, 127-132.

McClelland, J.L. and Rumelhart, D.E., An interactive activation model of context effects in letter perception: Part 1. An account of basic findings. Psychological Review, 1981, 88, 375-407.

Neisser, U. Cognitive psychology. New York: Appleton-Century-Crofts, 1967.

Pastore, R.E., Possible psychoacoustic factors in speech perception. In P.D. Eimas and J.L. Miller (Eds.) Perspectives on the study of speech. Hillsdale, New Jersey: Erlbaum, 1981.

Pisoni, D.B., Some current theoretical issues in speech perception. Cognition, 1981, 10, in press.

Rees, N.S., Saying more than we know: Is auditory processing disorder a meaningful concept? In R.W. Keith (Ed.) Central auditory and language disorders in children. Houston: College-Hill Press, 1981.

Remez, R.E., Adaptation of the category boundary between speech and non-speech: A case against feature detectors, Cognitive Psychology, 1979, 11, 38-57.

Remez, R.E., Rubin, P.E., Pisoni, D.B., and Carrell, T.D., Speech perception without traditional cues. Science, 1981, 212, 947-950.

Robinson, D.E. and Watson, C.S., Psychophysical methods in modern psychoacoustics. In J.V. Tobias (Ed.) Foundations of modern audiology, Volume 2. New York: Academic Press, 1972.

Schneider, B.A., Trehub, S.E. and Bull, D., The development of basic auditory processes in infants. Canadian Journal of Psychology, 1979, 33, 306-319.

Skinner, B.F., The behavior of organisms. New York: Appleton-Century, 1938.

Stevens, K.N., The potential role of property detectors in the perception of consonants. In G. Fant and M.A.A. Tatham

(Eds.), Auditory analysis and perception of speech. New York: Academic Press, 1975, 303-330.

Straight, H.S., Auditory versus articulatory phonological processes and their development in children. In G.H. Yeni-Komshian, J.F. Kavanagh, and C.A. Ferguson (Eds.), Child Phonology, Volume 1: Production. New York: Academic Press, 1980.

Strange, W. and Broen, P.A., Perception and Production of approximant consonants by three year-olds: A first study. In G.H. Yeni-Komshian, J.F. Kavanagh and C.A. Ferguson (Eds.), Child Phonology, Volume 2: Perception, New York: Academic Press, 1980.

Studdert-Kennedy, M., Speech perception. Language and Speech, 1980, 23, 45-65.

Tallal, P. and Stark, R.E., Speech perception of language-delayed children. In G.H. Yeni-Komshian, J.F. Kavanagh and C.A. Ferguson (Eds.), Child Phonology, Volume 2: Perception, New York: Academic Press, 1980.

Tallal, P., Stark, R., Kallman, C., and Mellits, D., Perceptual constancy for phonemic categories. Applied Psycholinguistics, 1980, 1, 49-64.

Trehub, S.E., Bull, D., and Schneider, B.A. Infant speech and nonspeech perception. In R.L. Schiefelbusch and D.D. Bricker (Eds.) Early Language: Acquisition and intervention. Baltimore: University Park Press, 1981(a).

Trehub, S.E., Bull, D., and Schneider, B.A., Infant's detection of speech in noise. Journal of Speech and Hearing Research, 1981, 24, 202-206(b).

Warren, R.M., Obusek, C.J., Farmer, R.M., and Warren, R.P. Auditory sequence: Confusion of patterns other than speech or music. Science, 1969, 164, 586-587.

Yeni-Komshian, G.H., Kavanagh, J.F. and Ferguson, C.A., Child Phonology. Volume 2: Perception. New York: Academic Press, 1980.

BIBLIOGRAPHY

Abramson, A., & Lisker, L. Discriminability along the voicing continuum: Cross-language tests. In Proceedings of the 6th International Congress of Phonetic Sciences (1967). Prague: Academia, 1970.

Armitage, S., Baldwin, B., & Vince, M. The fetal sound environment of sheep. Science, 1980, 208, 1173-1174.

Aslin, R.N., & Pisoni, D.B. Some developmental processes in speech perception. In G.H. Yeni-Komshian,J.P. Kavanagh & C.A. Ferguson (Eds.), Child phonology: Perception (Vol. 2). New York: Academic Press, 1980.

Aslin, R., Pisoni, D., & Jusczyk, P. Auditory development and speech perception in infancy. In P.H. Musson (Ed.), Carmichael's handbook of infant development, in press.

Atkinson, K.B., McWhinney, B., & Stoel, C. An experiment in the recognition of babbling. Papers and Reports on Child Language Development (No. 1). Stanford, 1970.

Austin, J. How to do things with words. Cambridge: Harvard University Press, 1962.

Babighian, G., Moushegian, G., Rupert, A., & Glorig, A. Central components of auditory fatigue. Some clinical implications. Proceedings of the Xth World Congress of Otorhinolaryngology, Excerpta Medica, 1973, 276, 95-96.

Baddeley, A.D. The psychology of memory. New York: Basic Books, 1976.

Barton, D. Phonemic perception in children. In G.H. Yeni-Komshian, J.F. Kavanagh & C.A. Ferguson (Eds.), Child phonology: Perception (Vol. 2). New York: Academic Press, 1980.

Bast, T., & Anson, B.J. The temporal bone and the ear. Springfield: Charles C Thomas, 1949.

Bates, E. Language and context: The acquisition of pragmatics. New York: Academic Press, 1976.

Bates, E., Benigini, L., Bretherton, I., Camaioni, L., &
Volterra, V. The emergence of symbols. New York:
Academic Press, 1979.

Bates, E., & MacWhinney, E. Functionalist approaches to grammar. In L. Gleitman & E. Wanner (Eds.), Language acquisition: The state of the art. New York: Cambridge University Press, in press.

Beebe, H. Deaf children can learn to hear. Talk, 1975, 75,
6-8.

Bench, J. Audio-frequency and audio-intensity discrimination
in the human neonate. International Audiology, 1969, 8
(4), 615-625.

Bench, J. The basics of infant hearing screening: why early
diagnosis? In S.E. Gerber & G.T. Mencher (Eds.), Early
diagnosis of hearing loss. New York: Grune & Stratton,
1978.

Bench, J. & Mentz, L. Stimulus complexity, state and infants'
auditory behavioral responses. British Journal of Disorders of Communication, 1975, 10, 52-60.

Bench, J., Collyer, J., Mentz, L., & Wilson, I. Studies in
infant behavioral audiometry: II. Six-week-old infants.
Audiology, 1976, 15, 302-314.

Berkeley, G. An essay toward a new theory of vision, 1709.

Bever, T. Some theoretical and empirical issues that arise if
we insist on distinguishing language and thought. Annals
of the New York Academy of Science, 1975, 263, 76-83.

Bickford, R., Jacobson, J., & Cody, D. Nature of averaged
evoked potentials to sound and other stimuli in man.
Annals of the New York Academy of Science, 1964, 112,
204-223.

Blackwell, P., Engen, E., Fischgrund, J.E., & Zarcadoolas,
C. Sentences and other systems: A language and learning
curriculum for hearing-impaired children. Washington,
D.C.: A.G. Bell Assoc., 1978.

Bloom, L.M. Language development: Form and function in emerging grammars. Cambridge, Mass.: MIT Press, 1970.

Blumenthal, A.L. Prompted recall of sentences. Journal of
    Verbal Learning and Verbal Behavior, 1967, 6, 203-206.

Blumstein, S.E. Speech perception: an overview. In G.H. Yeni-
    Komshian, J.F. Kavanagh & C.A. Ferguson (Eds.), Child
    phonology: Perception (Vol. 2). New York: Academic Press,
    1980.

Bordley, J., Ruben, R. & Lieberman, A. Human cochlear poten-
    tials. Laryngoscope, 1964, 74, 463-479.

Braine, M.D.S. The ontogeny of English phrase structure: the
    first phase. Language, 1963, 39, 1-13.

Bredberg, G. Cellular pattern and nerve supply of the human
    organ of Corti. Acta Otolaryngologica, 1968, 236.
    (Suppl.)

Bregman, A.S. Asking the 'what for' question in auditory
    perception. In M. Kubovy & J.R. Pomerantz (Eds.), Per-
    ceptual organization. Hillsdale, New Jersey: Lawrence
    Erlbaum Associates, 1981.

Broadbent, D.E. Perception and communication. Oxford: Perga-
    mon Press, 1958.

Brown, R.W. A first language: The early stages. Cambridge,
    Mass.: Harvard University Press, 1973.

Bruner, J.S. From communication to language: A psychological
    perspective. Cognition, 1975, 3, 255-287,

Bruner, J.S., Goodnow, J.J., & Austin, G.A. A study of think-
    ing. New York: John Wiley and Sons, 1956.

Bull, D., Schneider, B.A., & Trehub, S.E. The masking of
    octave-band noise by broad-spectrum noise: A comparison
    of infant and adult thresholds. Perception and Psycho-
    physics, 1981, 30, 101-106.

Bull, D., Trehub, S.E., & Schneider, B.A. A procedure for
    infant psychophysical testing. In preparation.

Bush, C.N., Edwards, M.L., Luckau, J.M., Stoel, C.M., Macken,
    M.A., & Peterson, J.D. On specifying a system for tran-
    scribing consonants in Child Language. Child Language
    Project, Committee on Linguistics. Stanford University,
    1973.

Carnes, A., Widen, G., & Viemeister, N. Noncategorical per-
    ception of stop consonants differing in VOT. Journal of
    the Acoustical Society of America, 1977, 62, 961-970.

Chomsky, N. Syntactic structures. The Hague: Mouton, 1957.

Chomsky, N. Aspects of the theory of syntax. Cambridge, Mass.:
    MIT Press, 1965.

Clark, E.V. What's in a word? On the child's acquisition of
    semantics in his first language. In T.E. Moore (Ed.),
    Cognitive development and the acquisition of Language.
    New York: Academic Press, 1973.

Clark, E.V. From gesture to word: on the natural history of
    deixis in language acquisition. In J.S. Bruner & A.
    Garton (Eds.) Human growth and development: Wolfson
    College Lectures, 1976. Oxford: Oxford University Press,
    1978.

Cohen, S., Glass, D.C. & Singer, J.E. Apartment noise, aud-
    itory discrimination and reading ability in children.
    Journal of Experimental Social Psychology, 1973, 9,
    407-422.

Colburn, H.S., & Durlach, J.I. Models of binaural interac-
    tion. In E.C. Carterette & M.P. Friedman (Eds.), Hand-
    book of perception: Hearing (Vol. 4). New York: Academic
    Press, 1978.

Cole, R.A., & Scott, B. Toward a theory of speech perception.
    Psychological Review, 1974, 81, 348-374.

Cone, B.K. Auditory evoked potentials for pediatric evalua-
    tions. Audiology and Hearing Education, 1980, 6(3),
    7-11.

Crowder, R.G., & Morton, J. Precategorical acoustic storage
    (PAS). Perception and Psychophysics, 1969, 5, 365-373.

Crowell, D.H., Jones, R.H., Nakagawa, J.K., & Kapuniai, L.E.
    Heart rate response of human new borns to modulated pure
    tones. Proceedings of the Royal Society of Medicine,
    971, 64, 474.

Cruttenden, A. A Phonetic Study of Babbling. British Journal
    of Dis. of Communication, 1970, 5, 110-118.

Curtiss, S. Linguistic Department, University of California,
    Los Angeles. Personal communication, 1981.

Cutting, J.E., & Rosner, B.S. Categories and boundaries in
    speech and music. Perception and Psychophysics, 1974,
    16, 564-570.

de Boysson Bardies, B., Sagart, L., & Bacri, N. Phonetic
    analysis of late babbling: A case study of a French
    child. Journal of Child Language, 1981, 8, 511-524.

DeCasper, A., & Fifer, W. Of human bonding: Newborns prefer
    their mothers' voices. Science, 1980, 208, 1174-1176.

Deol, M.S. The abnormalities of the inner ear in Kreisler
    mice. Journal of Embryology and Experimental Morphology,
    1964, 12, 475-490.

Deol, M.S. Influence of the neural tube on the differentia-
    tion of the inner ear in the mammalian embryo. Nature,
    1966, 209, 219-220.

Deol, M.S. Genetic malformations of the inner ear in mouse
    and man. In R.J. Gorlin (Ed.), Morphogenesis and mal-
    formation of the ear. Birth defects: Original article
    series (Vol. XVI, No. 4). New York: Allan R. Liss, Inc.,
    1980.

Dore, J. A pragmatic description of early language develop-
    ment. Journal of Psycholinguistic Research, 1974, 4,
    343-350.

Downs, M.P., & Sterritt, G.M. Identification audiometry for
    neonates: a preliminary report. Journal of Auditory
    Research, 1964, 4, 69-80.

Durlach, N.I., & Colburn, H.S. Binaural and spatial hearing.
    In E.C. Carterette & M.P. Friedman (Eds.), Handbook of
    perception: Hearing (Vol. 4). New York: Academic Press,
    1978.

Eady, S. The onset of language-specific patterning in infant
    vocalization. Unpublished master's thesis, University of
    Ottawa, 1980.

Eilers, R.E. Infant speech perception: history and mystery.
    In G.H. Yeni-Komshian, J.F. Kavanagh & C.A. Ferguson
    (Eds.), Child phonology: Perception (Vol. 2). New York:

Academic Press, 1980.

Eilers, R.E., Oller, D.K., & Benito-Garcia, C.R. The acquisition of voicing contrasts in Spanish and English-learning infants and children: A longitudinal study. Paper
presented at the Acoustical Society of America Convention, Miami Beach, 1981.

Eimas, P., Auditory and linguistic processing of cues for
place of articulation by infants. Perception and Psychophysics, 1974, 16, 513-521.

Eimas, P. Auditory and phonetic coding of the cues for
speech: Discrimination of the /r-l/ distinction by
young infants. Perception and Psychophysics, 1975, 18,
341-347.

Eimas, P., Siqueland, E.R., Jusczyk, P., & Vigorito, D.J.
Speech perception in infants. Science, 1971, 171, 303-
306.

Eimas, P., & Miller, J.L. Effects of selective adaptation on
the perception of speech and visual patterns: evidence
for feature detectors. In R.D. Walk & H.L. Pick (Eds.),
Perception and experience. New York: Plenum Press, 1978.

P.D. Eimas, & J.L. Miller (Eds.), Perspectives on the study
of speech. Hillsdale, New Jersey: Lawrence Erlbaum
Associates, 1981.

Eimas, P., & Tartter, V. On the development of speech perception: Mechanisms and analogies. In H. Reese & L.
Lipsitt (Eds.), Advances in child development and behavior (Vol. 13). New York: Academic Press, 1979.

Eimas, P.D., Tartter, V.C., & Miller, J.L. Dependency during
the processing of speech. In P.D. Eimas & J.L. Miller
(Eds.), Perspectives on the study of speech. Hillsdale,
New Jersey: Lawrence Erlbaum Associates, 1981.

Eisenberg, R.B. Auditory behavior in the human neonate: functional properties of sound and their ontogenic implications. International Audiology, 1969, 8, 34-45.

Eisenberg, R.B. Pediatric audiology: shadow or substance?
Journal of Auditory Research, 1971, 11, 148-153.

Eisenberg, R.B. Auditory competence in early life: The roots of communicative behavior. Baltimore, MD: University Park Press, 1976.

Elliott, L.L. Performance of children aged 9 to 17 years on a test of speech intelligibility in noise using sentence material with controlled word predictability. Journal of the Acoustical Society of America, 1979, 66, 651-653.

Elliott, L.L., & Katz, D.R. Children's Pure-Tone Detection. Journal of the Acoustical Society of America, 1980, 67, 343-344.

Engel, R., & Young, N.B. Calibrated pure tone audiograms in normal neonates based on evoked electroencephalic responses. Neuropädiatrie, 1969, 1, 149-160.

Erber, N. Auditory, visual, and auditory-visual recognition of consonants by children with normal and impaired hearing. Journal of Speech and Hearing Research, 1972, 2, 413-422.

Erber, N. Auditory-visual perception of speech. Journal of Speech and Hearing Disorders, 1975, 40, 481-492.

Falk, S.A., Cook, R.O., Haseman, J.K., & Sanders, G.M. Noise-induced inner ear damage in newborn and adult guinea pigs. Laryngoscope, 1974, 83, 444-453.

Falk, S.A., & Farmer, J.C. Incubator noise and possible deafness. Archives of Otolaryngology, 1973, 97, 385-387.

Feinmesser, M., & Tell, L. Progress report: Evaluation of methods of detecting hearing impariment in infancy and early childhood. Hadassah Hospital, Jerusalem, Israel, 1971, V.S.P.H.S.-M.C.H.S. Project 06-48D-Z.

Ferguson, C.A. Baby talk in six languages. American Anthropology, 1964, 66, 103-114.

Fernald, A. Four-month-olds prefer to listen to 'Motherese'. Paper presented at the Society for Research in Child Development, Boston, 1981.

Fernald, A., & Kuhl, P. Fundamental frequency as an acoustic determinant of infant preference for 'Motherese'. Paper presented at the Society for Research in Child Development, Boston, 1981.

Fernald, A., & Simon, T. Expanded intonation contours in mothers' speech to newborns. In preparation.

Fillmore, C.J. The case for case. In E. Bach & R.T. Harms
    (Eds.), Universals in linguistic theory. New York: Holt,
    Rinehart & Winston, 1968.

Fischer, K.W. A theory of cognitive development. Psychologi-
    cal Review, 1980, 87, 477-531.

Fitzgerald, E. Straight language for the deaf. Washington,
    D.C.: The Volta Bureau, 1949.

Flavell, J.H. The developmental psychology of Jean Piaget.
    New York: Van Nostrand, 1963.

Fleischer, K. Untersuchungen zur entwicklung der
    innenohrfunktion. Z. Laryng. Rhinol. Otolaryngol., 1955,
    34, 733.

Franklin, B. Audiometric testing using narrow speech bands.
    Paper presented at the International Congress on Educa-
    tion of the Deaf. Hamburg, 1980.

Franklin, B. Newborn responses to acoustic stimuli. Paper
    presented at the 102nd meeting of the Acoustical Society
    of America. Miami Beach, 1981.

Fraser, G.R. The causes of profound deafness in childhood.
    London: Bailliere-Tindal, 1976.

Friedlander, B.Z. Receptive language development in infancy.
    Merrill-Palmer Quarterly, 1970, 16, 7-51.

Galambos, R., Makeig, S., & Talmachoff, P. A 40-Hz auditory
    potential recorded from the human scalp. Proceedings of
    the National Academy of Science, 1981, 78, 2643-2647.

Gardi, J., & Bledgoe, S. Elucidation of the origins of the
    middle components (8-25 msec) of the AER in the cat
    using a serial ablation technique. Paper presented at
    the Symposium of the International Electric Response
    Audiometry Study Group, Santa Barbara, 1979.

Geisler, C., Frishkopf, L., & Rosenblith, W. Extracranial
    responses to acoustic clicks in man. Science, 1958,
    128, 1210-1211.

Gerber, S.E. Neonatal auditory testing: A review. In G.C.
    Cunningham (Ed.), Conference on newborn hearing screen-

ing. Berkeley: California State Department of Public
Health, 1971.

Gerber, S.E., Jones, B.L., & Costello, J.M. Behavioral measures. In S.E. Gerber (Ed.), Audiometry in infancy. New
York: Grune & Stratton, Inc., 1977.

Gerber, S.E., Lima, C.G., & Copriviza, K.L. Auditory arousal
in preterm infants. Scandinavian Audiology, in press.

Gerber, S.E., & Mencher, G.T. Arousal responses of neonates
to wide band and narrow band noise. Paper presented at
the Annual Convention of the American Speech-Language-
Hearing Association, Atlanta, 1979.

Gerber, S.E., Mendel, M.I., & Goller, M. Progressive hearing
loss subsequent to congenital cytomegalovirus infection.
Human Communication, 1979, 4, 232-233.

Gerber, S.E., & Milner, P. The transitivity of loudness level.
Journal of the Audio Engineering Society, 1971, 19, 656-
659.

Gerber, S.E., Mulac, A., & Swain, B.J. Idiosyncratic cardiovascular response of human neonates to acoustic stimuli.
The Journal of the American Audiology Society, 1976, 1
(5), 185-191

Gibson, J.J. The senses considered as perceptual systems.
Boston: Houghton Mifflin, 1966.

Gibson, J.J., & Gibson, E.J. Perceptual learning-differentiation or enrichment? Psychological Review, 1955, 62,
32-41.

Goff, W., Allison, T., Lyons, W., et al. Origins of short
latency auditory evoked response components in man. In
J. Desmedt (Ed.), Auditory Evoked Potentials in Man.
Basel: Karger, 1977.

Goldstein, R., & McRandle, C.C. Middle components of the
averaged electroencephalic response to clicks in neo-
nates. In S.K. Hirsh, D.H. Eldridge, I.J. Hirsh & S.R.
Silverman (Eds.), Hearing and Davis: Essays honoring
Hallowell Davis. St. Louis, Mo.: Washington University
Press, 1976.

Griffiths, C. Auditory training in the first year of life.

In Proceedings of the International conference on oral
education of the deaf (Vol. 1). Washington, D.C.: A.G.
Bell Associates, 1967.

Guilford, J.P. Psychometric methods (2nd ed.). New York:
McGraw-Hill Book Co., 1954.

Haggard, M. Do we want a theory of speech perception? Paper
presented at the Research Conference on Speech-Process-
ing Aids for the Deaf, Gallaudet College, Washington,
D.C., May, 1977.

Halliday, M. Learning how to mean. London: Edward Arnold,
1975.

Hardy, J.D., Hardy, W.G., & Hardy, M.P. Some problems in neonatal screening. Trans. Amer. Acad. Ophthalmol. Otolaryngol., 1970, 74, 1229-1235.

Harker. L.A., Hosick, E., Voots, R.J., & Mendel, M.I. Influence of succinylcholine on middle component auditory
evoked potentials. Archives of Otolaryngology, 1977,
103, 133-137.

Harris, S., & Almqvist, B. ABR in operatively verified
cerebello-pontine angle tumors. Scandinavian Symposium
on Brain Stem Response, Scandinavian Audiology, 1981,
Suppl. 13, 113-114.

Hawkins, J.E., Jr., & Stevens, S.S. The masking of pure tones
and of speech by white noise. Journal of the Acoustical
Society of America, 1950, 22, 6-13.

Hecox, K., & Galambos, R. Brain stem auditory evoked responses in human infants and adults. Archives of Otolaryngology, 1974, 99, 30-33.

Held, H. Untersuchungen über den feineren Bau des
Ohrlabyrinthes der Wirbelthiere: II Zur
Entwicklungsgeschichte des Cortischen Organs und der
Macula Acustica bei Sangethieren und Vogeln. Abhandl. d.
math. phys. k.d.k. Sachs. Gesellsch.d. Wissensch.,
(Leipzig) 1909, 31, 193-293.

Hertwig, P. Die geneses der hirn und gehörganmissifildungen
bei röntgenmutierten Kreisler-mausen. Z. Mensch. Vereb.
Konst., 1944, 28, 327-354.

Hillenbrand, J. Perceptual Organization of Speech Sounds by Young Infants. Unpublished Doctoral dissertation, University of Washington, 1980.

Horiuchi, K. Auditory middle latency response. Otolaryngology J.Japan, 1976, 79, 1549-1558.

Hoversten, G.H., & Moncur, J.P. Stimuli and intensity factors in testing infants. Journal of Speech and Hearing Research, 1960, 12, 687-702.

Huizing, H. Auditory training. Acta Oto-laryngologica, 1951, 100, 158-163. (Suppl.)

Hutt, S.J., Hutt, C., Lenard, H.G., von Bernuth, H., & Muntjewerff, W.J. Auditory responsivity in the human neonate. Nature, 1968, 218, 888-890.

Jakobson, R. Kindersprache, Aphasie und Allgemeine Lautgesetze. Uppsala: Almqvist and Wiksell, 1941.

James, W. What pragmatism means-pragmatism: A new name for some old ways of thinking. New York: Longmans, Green, and Co., 1907.

Jewett, D.L., & Williston, J.S. Auditory-evoked far fields averaged from the scalp of humans. Brain, 1971, 94, 681-696.

Johansson, B., Wedenberg, E., & Westin, B. Measurement of tone response by the human foetus. Acta Oto-laryngologica, 1970, 57, 1229-1235.

Joint Committee on Infant Hearing Screening. Statement of November 1970. Asha, 1971, 12, 79.

Joint Committee on Infant Hearing Screening. Supplementary statement, July 1, 1972. Asha, 1974, 16, 160.

Joint Committee on Infant Hearing. Position Statement, 1982. Pediatrics, 1982, 70(3), 496-497.

Jones, M.R. Time, our lost dimension: toward a new theory of perception, attention, and memory. Psychological Review, 1976, 83,323-355.

Jusczyk, P.W. Infant speech perception: A critical appraisal. In P.D. Eimas & J.L. Miller (Eds.), Perspectives on the study of speech. Hillsdale, New Jersey: Lawrence Erlbaum Associates, 1981.

Jusczyk, P.W., Rosner, B.S., Cutting, J.E., Foard, C.F., & Smith, L.B. Categorical perception of non-speech sounds by two-month old infants. Perception and Psychophysics, 1977, 21, 50-54.

Just, M.A., & Carpenter, P.A. A theory of reading: from eye fixations to comprehension. Psychological Review, 1980, 87, 329-354.

Kaga, K., Hink, R., Shinoda, Y., & Suzuki, J. Origin of a middle latency component in cats. Paper presented at the Symposium of the International Electric Response Audiometry Study Group, Santa Barbara, 1979.

Katz, J. The staggered spondaic word test. In R.W. Keith (Ed.), Central auditory dysfunction. New York: Grune & Stratton, 1977.

Kent, R. Articulatory-acoustic perspectives on speech development. In R. Stark (Ed.), Language behavior in infancy and early childhood. New York: Elsevier, 1980.

Klima, E.S., & Bellugi, U. Syntactic regularities in the speech of children. In J. Lyons & R.J. Wales (Eds.), Psycholinguistics papers. Edinburgh: Edinburgh University Press, 1966.

Kuhl, P. Speech perception in early infancy: The acquisition of speech sound categories. In S. Hirsh, D. Eldredge, I. Hirsh & S. Silverman (Eds.), Hearing and Davis: Essays honoring Hallowell Davis. St. Louis: Washington University Press, 1976.

Kuhl, P. The perception of speech in early infancy. In N. Lass (Ed.), Speech and language: Advances in basic research and practice. New York: Academic Press, 1979a.

Kuhl, P. Speech perception in early infancy: Perceptual constancy for spectrally dissimilar vowel categories. Journal of the Acoustical Society of America, 1979b, 66, 1668-1679.

Kuhl, P. Models and mechanisms in speech perception: Species comparisons provide further contributions. Brain, Behavior Evolution, 1979c., 16, 374-408.

Kuhl, P.K. Perceptual constancy for speech-sound categories
     in early infancy. In G.H. Yeni-Komshian, J.F. Kavanagh
     & C.A. Ferguson (Eds.), Child phonology: Perception
     (Vol. 2). New York: Academic Press, 1980.

Kuhl, P. Perception of speech and sound in early infancy. In
     P. Salapatek & L.B. Cohen (Eds.) Handbook of infant per-
     ception. New York: Academic Press, in press.

Kuhl, P. Constancy, categorization, and perceptual organiza-
     tion for speech and sound in early infancy. In J. Mehler
     (Ed.), Neonatal cognition: Beyond the blooming confu-
     sion. Hillsdale, NJ: Lawrence Erlbaum Assoc., in press.

Kuhl, P. Perception of auditory equivalence classes for
     speech in early infancy. Infant behavior and develop-
     ment, in press.

Kuhl, P., & Miller, J. Speech perception in the chinchilla:
     voiced-voiceless distinction in alveolar plosive con-
     sonants. Science, 1975, 190, 69-72.

Kuhl, P., & Meltzoff, A. The bimodal perception of speech in
     infancy. Science, in press.

Kuhl, P., & Miller, J.D. Speech perception by the chinchilla:
     identification functions for synthetic VOT stimuli.
     Journal of the Acoustical Society of America, 1978,
     63, 905-917.

Kuhl, P., & Padden, D. Speech discrimination by macaques:
     auditory constraints on the evolution of language.
     Perception and psychophysics, in press. (a)

Kuhl, P., & Padden, D. Speech discrimination by macaques:
     Enhanced discrimination at the phonetic boundaries be-
     tween speech-sound categories. Journal of the Acousti-
     cal Society of America, in press. (b)

Kupperman, G.L., & Mendel, M.I. Threshold of the early com-
     ponents of the averaged electroencephalic response de-
     termined with tone pips and clicks during drug-induced
     sleep. Audiology, 1974, 13, 379-390.

Kyle, J.G. The study of auditory deprivation from birth.
     British Journal of Audiology, 1978, 12, 37-39.

Lach, R., Ling, D., Ling, A.H., & Ship, N. Early speech de-

velopment in deaf infants. American Annals of the Deaf,
1970, 115, 522-526.

Lenneberg, E.H. Biological foundations of language. New York:
John Wiley & Sons, Inc., 1967.

Lewis, M.M. Infant speech: A study of the beginnings of language. New York: Harcourt, Brace and World, 1936.

Li, C.W., Van De Water, T.R., & Ruben, R.J. The fate mapping
of the eleventh and twelfth day mouse otocyst: an 'in
vitro' study of the sites of origin of the embryonic
inner ear sensory structures. Journal of Morphology,
1978, 157, 249-268.

Liberman, A.M., Cooper, F.S., Shankweiler, D.P., & Studdert-
Kennedy, M. Perception of the speech code. Psychological
Review, 1967, 74, 431-461.

Licklider, J.C.R. Basic correlates of the auditory stimulus.
In S.S. Stevens (Ed.), Handbook of experimental psychology. New York: John Wiley and Sons, 1951.

Ling, A.H. Schedules of development in audition, speech,
langauge, communication for hearing impaired infants &
their parents. Washington, D.C.: A.G. Bell Assoc., 1977.

Ling, D. The education and general background of children
with defective hearing in the borough of Reading. Unpublished research associateship thesis, Cambridge
University Institute of Education, England, 1959.

Ling, D. Response validity in auditory tests of newborn infants. Laryngoscope, 1972, 82, 376-380.

Ling, D. Recent developments affecting the education of
hearing-impaired children. Public Health Reviews,
1975, 4, 117-152.

Ling, D. Speech and the hearing impaired child: Theory &
practice. Washington, D.C.: A.G. Bell Assoc., 1976.

Ling, D., & Ling, A.H. Aural habilitation: The foundation of
verbal learning in hearing-impaired children. Washington, D.C.: A.G. Bell Assoc., 1978.

Ling, D., Ling, A.H., & Doehring, D.G. Stimulus, response and
observer variables in the auditory screening of newborn

infants. Journal of Speech and Hearing Research, 1970,
13(1), 9-18.

Ling, D., Ling, A.H., & Jacobson, C. Detection and treatment
of deafness in early infancy. Canadian Family Physician,
1968, 14, 47-52.

Ling, D., & Milne, M.F. The development of speech in hearing-
impaired children. In F.H. Bess, B.A. Freeman & J.S.
Sinclair (Eds.), Amplification in education. Washington,
D.C.: A.G. Bell Assoc., 1981.

Lisker, L. Rapid vs. rabid: A catalogue of acoustic features
that may cue the distinctions. Haskins Laboratory Status
Report on Speech Research, 1978, SR-54, 127-132.

Lisker, L., & Abramson, A. A cross-language study of voicing
in initial stops: Acoustical measurements. Word, 1964,
20, 384-422.

Lorento de No, R. Etudes sur l'anatomie at la physiologie du
labyrinthe de l'orielle et du VIII: e nerf. Trab. Inst.
Cajal Invest Biol., 1926, 24, 43.

Luterman, D. Counseling parents of hearing-impaired children.
Boston: Little, Brown & Co., 1979.

Lynip, A.W. The use of magnetic devices in the collection and
analysis of the preverbal utterances of an infant.
Genetic Psychology Monographs, 1951, 44, 221-262.

Madell, J.R., & Goldstein, R. Relation between loudness and
the amplitude of the early components of the averaged
electroencephalic response. Journal of Speech and Hearing Research, 1972, 14, 134-141.

Mason, L.A. Neonates' responses to loudness-balanced wide and
narrow band acoustic stimuli. Unpublished Master's
thesis, University of California, Santa Barbara, 1981.

McClelland, J.L., & Rumelhart, D.R. An interactive activation
model of context effects in letter perception: part 1.
An account of basic findings. Psychological Review,
1981, 88, 375-407.

McFarland, W.H., Vivion, M.C., & Goldstein, R. Middle components of the AER to tone-pips in normal-hearing-impair-
ed subjects. Journal of Speech and Hearing Research,

1977, 20, 781-798.

McGurk, K., & MacDonald, J. Hearing lips and seeing voices. Nature, 1976, 264, 746-748.

McNeill, D. Developmental psycholinguistics. In F. Smith & G.A. Miller (Eds.), The genesis of language. Cambridge, Mass.: MIT Press, 1966.

McRandle, C.C., Smith, M.A., & Goldstein, R. Early averaged electroencephalic responses to clicks in neonates. Annals of Otology, Rhinology and Laryngology, 1974, 83, 695-702.

Meltzoff, A. Imitation, intermodal coordination, and representation in early infancy. In G. Butterworth (Ed.), Infancy and epistemology. London: Harvester Press, 1981.

Meltzoff, A., & Borton, T. Intermodal matching by human neonates. Nature, 1979, 282, 403-404.

Meltzoff, A., & Moore, K. Imitation of facial and manual gestures by human neonates. Science, 1977, 198, 75-78.

Meltzoff, A., & Moore, K. Human newborns imitate adult facial gestures. Child development, in press.

Mencher, G.T. A program for neonatal hearing screening. Audiology, 1974, 13, 9-18.

G.T. Mencher (Ed.), Early identification of hearing loss. Basel: S. Karger, 1976.

Mencher, G.T., Derbyshire, A.J., McCulloch, B., & Dethlefs, R. Observer bias as a factor in neonatal hearing screening. Paper presented at the Annual Convention of the American Speech and Hearing Association, Detroit, 1973.

Mencher, G.T., & Mencher, L.S. Auditory pathologies in infancy. Paper presented at the Conference on Auditory Development in Infancy, Erindale symposium, Toronto, 1981.

Mendel, M.I. Infant responses to recorded sounds. Journal of Speech and Hearing Research, 1968, 11, 811-816.

Mendel, M.I. Electroencephalic tests of hearing. In S.E. Gerber (Ed.), Audiometry in infancy. New York: Grune &

Stratton, 1977.

Mendel, M.I. Clinical use of primary cortical responses.
Audiology, 1980, 19, 1-15.

Mendel, M.I., Adkinson, C.D., & Harker, L.A. Middle components of the auditory evoked potentials in infants.
Annals of Otology, Rhinology and Laryngology, 1977, 86,
293-299.

Mendel, M.I., & Goldstein, R. The effect of test conditions
on the early components of the averaged electroencephalic response. Journal of Speech and Hearing Research,
1969, 12, 344-350.

Mendel, M.I., & Goldstein, R. Early components of the averaged electroencephalic response to constant level clicks
during all-night sleep. Journal of Speech and Hearing
Research, 1971, 14, 829-840.

Mendel, M.I., & Hosick, E.C. Effects of secobarbital on the
early components of the auditory evoked potentials.
Revue de Laryngologie, 1975, 96, 178-184.

Mendelson, T., & Salamy, A. Maturational effects on the middle components of the averaged electroencephalic response. Journal of Speech and Hearing Research, 1981,
24, 140-144.

Menyuk, P. The role of distinctive features in children's
acquisition of phonology. Journal of Speech and Hearing Research, 1968, 11, 138-146.

Miller, G.A., & McKean, K.E. A chronometric study of some relations between sentences. Quarterly Journal of Experimental Psychology, 1964, 16, 297-308.

Miller, J. Effects of speaking rate on segmental distinctions. In P. Eimas & J. Miller (Eds.), Perspectives on
the study of speech. Hillsdale, NJ: Lawrence Erlbaum
Assoc., 1981.

Mills, J.H. Noise and children: A review of literature.
Journal of the Acoustical Society of America, 1975, 58,
767-779.

Montgomery, G.W. The relationship of oral skills to manual
communication in profoundly deaf adolescents. American

Annals of the Deaf, 1966, 111, 557-565.

Moore, J.M., Thompson, G., & Thompson, M. Auditory localization of infants as a function of reinforcement conditions. Journal of Speech and Hearing Research, 1975, 40,
29-34.

Moore, J.M., & Wilson, W.R. Visual reinforcement audimetry
(VRA) with infants. In S.E. Gerber & G.T. Mencher (Eds.),
Early diagnosis of hearing loss. New York: Grune &
Stratton, Inc., 1980.

Moores, D.F. Educating the deaf. Boston, Mass.: Houghton,
Mifflin Co., 1978.

Moses, K.L., & Van Hecke-Wulatin, M. The socio-emotional
impact of infant deafness: a counselling model. In G.T.
Mencher & S.E. Gerber (Eds.), Early management of hearing loss. New York: Grune & Stratton, 1981.

Muir, D., & Field, J. Newborn infants orient to sounds. Child
Development, 1979, 50, 431-436.

Muir, D., Abraham, W., Forbes, B., & Harris, L. The ontogenesis of an auditory localization response from birth to
four months of age. Canadian Journal of Psychology,
1979, 33, 320-333.

Murai, J. The sounds of infants: their phonemicization and
symbolization. Studia Phonologica, 1963, 3, 17-34.

Murphy, K.P. Development of hearing in babies. Hearing News,
1961, 29, 9-11.

Nakazima, S.A. A comparative study of the speech developments
of Japanese and American English in childhood. Studia
Phonologica, 1962, 2, 27-39.

Neisser, U. Cognitive Psychology. New York: Appleton-Century-
Crofts, 1967.

Nelson, C. Individual differences in language development:
implications for development and language. Developmental
Psychology, 1981, 17, 170-187.

Netsell, R. The acquisition of speech motor control: A perspective with directions for research. In R. Stark (Ed.),

Language Behavior in Infancy and Early Childhood. New York: Elsevier, 1980.

Northern, J.L., & Downs, M.P. Hearing in Children (2nd ed.). The Williams & Wilkins Company: Baltimore, 1978.

Nozza, R.J. Detection of pure tones in quiet and in noise by infants and adults. Unpublished doctoral dissertation, University of Washington, 1981.

Oller, D.K. Infant vocalizations and the development of speech. Allied Health and Behavioral Sciences, 1978, 1, 523-549.

Oller, D.K. The emergence of the sounds of speech in infancy. In G. Yeni-Komshian, C. Ferguson & J. Kavanagh (Eds.), Child phonology. New York: Academic Press, 1980.

Oller, D.K. Infant vocalizations: Exploration and reflexivity. In R.E. Stark (Ed.), Language behavior in infancy and early childhood. New York: Elsevier: North Holland Publishing Co., 1981.

Oller, D.K., & Eilers, R.E. Phonetic expectation and transcription validity. Phonetica, 1975, 31, 288-304.

Oller, D.K., & Eilers, R.E. Similarities of babbling in Spanish and English-learning babies. Journal of Child Langauge, in press.

Oller, D.K., Wieman, L.A., Doyle, W., & Ross, C. Infant babbling and speech. Journal of Child Language, 1975, 3, 1-11.

Olney, R.L., & Scholnick, E.K. Adult judgments of age and linguistic differences in infant vocalization. Journal of Child Language, 1976, 3, 145-156.

Pastore, R.E. Possible psychoacoustic factors in speech perception. In P.D. Eimas & J.L. Miller (Eds.), Perspectives on the study of speech. Hillsdale, New Jersey: Lawrence Erlbaum Associates, 1981.

Peltzman, P., Kitterman, J.A., Ostwald, P.F., Manchester, D., & Health, L. Effects of incubator noise on human hearing. Journal of Auditory Research, 1970, 10, 335-339.

Piaget, J. The language and thought of the child. London:

Routledge and Kegan Paul Ltd., 1926.

Piaget, J. The construction of reality in the child. New
York: Basic Books, 1954.

Picton, T.W. The strategy of evoked potential audiometry. In
S.E. Gerber & G.T. Mencher (Eds.), Early diagnosis of
hearing loss. New York: Grune & Stratton, Inc., 1978.

Picton, T.W., & Hillyard, S.A. Human auditory evoked potentials. II. effects of attention. Electroencephalography
and Clinical Neurophysiology, 1974, 36, 191-200.

Picton, T.W., Hillyard, S.A., & Krausz, H.I. et al. Human
auditory evoked potentials. I. evaluation of components.
Electroencephalography and Clinical Neurophysiology,
1974, 36, 179-190.

Picton, T., & Smith A. The practice of evoked potential audiometry. Otolaryngology Clinics of North America, 1978,
11, 263-281.

Picton, T.W., Woods, D., & Baribeau-Braun, J. et al. Evoked
potential audiometry. Journal of Otolaryngology, 1977,
6, 90-119.

Pierce, C. How to Make Ideas Clear. Popular Science Monthly,
1978, 12, 286-302.

Pisoni, D.E. Some current theoretical models in speech perception. Cognition, 1981, 10, 249-259.

Pollack, D. Acoupedics: a uni-sensory approach to auditory
training. Volta Review, 1964, 66, 400-409.

Preston, M.S., Yeni-Komshian, G., & Stark, R.E. Voicing in
initial stop consonants produced by children in the prelinguistic period from different language communities.
Johns Hopkins University School of Medicine, Annual Report of Neurocommunications Lab., 1967, No. 2: 305-323.

Price, G.R. Loss in cochlear microphonic sensitivity in young
cat ears exposed to intense sound. Journal of the Acoustical Society of America, 1972, 51, 104(a).

Reed, N., Hirsh, I., & Goldstein, R. Maturation of early and
middle component AERs in infants. Paper presented at the
Annual Convention of the American Speech-Language-Hearing

Association, Detroit, 1980.

Rees, N.S. Saying more than we know: is auditory processing disorder a meaningful concept? In R.W. Keith (Ed.), Central auditory and language disorders in children. Houston: College-Hill Press, 1981.

Remez, R.E. Adaptation of the category boundary between speech and non-speech: A case against feature detectors. Cognitive Psychology, 1979, 11, 38-57.

Remez, R.E., Rubin, P.E., Pisoni, D.B., & Carrell, T.D. Speech perception without traditional cues. Science, 1981, 212, 947-950.

Repp, B. Categorical perception: Issues, methods, findings. In N. Lass (Ed.), Speech and language: Advances in basic research and practice. New York: Academic Press, in press.

Retzius, M.G. Das Gehörorgan der Wirbelthiere. Stockholm: Samson and Wallin, 1881-1884.

Riesen, A.H. Sensory deprivation. Progress in Physiological Psychology, 1966, 1, 117-147.

Robinson, D.E., & Watson, C.S. Psychophysical methods in modern psycho-acoustics. In J.V. Tobias (Ed.), Foundations of modern audiology (Vol. 2). New York: Academic Press, 1972.

Ruben, R.J. Development of the inner ear of the mouse: A radioautographic study of terminal mitoses. Acta Otolaryngologica, 1967, Suppl., 220, 1-44.

Ruben, R.J. Development and cell kinetics for the Kreisler (kr/kr) mouse. Laryngoscope, 1973, 83, 1440-1468.

Ruben, R.J., & Kruger, B. Hearing loss in the elderly. In R. Katzman & R. Terry (Eds.), Neurology of aging. F.A. Davis & Co. Book in preparation.

Ruben, R.J., & Rapin, I. Plasticity of the developing auditory system. Annals of Otology, Rhinology and Laryngology, 1980, 89, 303-311.

Russell, W.K., Quigley, S.P., & Power, D.J. Linguistics and deaf children. Washington: A.G. Bell Assoc., 1976.

Salamy, A., & McKean, C.M. Postnatal development of human
    brainstem potentials during the first year of life.
    Electroencephalography and Clinical Neurophysiology,
    1976, 40, 418-426.

Schneider, B.A., Trehub, S.E., & Bull, D. The development of
    basic auditory processes in infants. Canadian Journal of
    Psychology, 1979, 33, 306-310.

Schulman, C.A., & Wade, G. The use of heart rate in the aud-
    iological evaluation of nonverbal children. Part II.
    Clinical trials on an infant population. Neuropädiatrie,
    1970, 2, 197-205.

Scott, J.P., & Marston, M.V. Critical periods affecting the
    development of normal and maladjustive social behavior
    in puppies. Journal of Genetic Psychology, 1950, 77,
    25-60.

Searle, J. Speech acts: An essay in the philosophy of lan-
    guage. New York: Cambridge University Press, 1969.

Shankweiler, D., Strange, W., & Verbrugge, R. Speech and the
    problem of perceptual constancy. In R. Shaw & J.
    Bransford (Eds.), Perceiving, acting and knowing:
    Toward an ecological psychology. Cambridge: Cambridge
    University Press, 1977.

Sher, A.E. The embryonic and postnatal development of the
    inner ear of the mouse. Acta Otolaryngologica, Suppl.,
    1971, 284, 1-77.

Simmons, R.B., & Russ, F.N. Automated newborn hearing screen-
    ing, the Crib-o-gram. Archives of Otolaryngology, 1974,
    101, 1-7.

Skinner, B.F. The behavior of organisms. New York: Appleton-
    Century, 1938.

Snow, C., & Ferguson, C. Talking to children: Language input
    and acquisition. Cambridge University Press, 1978.

Sparks, D., Kuhl, P., Edmonds, A., & Gray, G. Investigating
    the MESA (Multipoint Electrotactile Speech Aid): The
    transmission of segmental features of speech. Journal
    of the Acoustical Society of America, 1978, 63, 246-257.

Spelke, E. Infants' intermodal perception of events. Cognitive Psychology, 1976, 8, 553-560.

Spelke, E. Perceiving biomodally specified events in infancy.
Developmental Psychology, 1979, 15, 626-636.

Starr, A., & Achor, J. Auditory brainstem responses in neuro-
logical disease. Archives of Neurology, 1975, 32, 761-
768.

Stern, D. The first relationship: Mother and infant. Cambridge: Harvard University Press, 1977.

Stern, D., Jaffe, J., Beebe, B., & Bennett, S. Vocalizing in
unison and in alternation: Two modes of communication in
the mother-infant dyad. Annals of the New York Academy
of Sciences, 1975, 263, 89-100.

Stevens, K.N. The potential role of property detectors in the
perception of consonants. In G. Fant & M.A.A. Tatham
(Eds.), Auditory analysis and perception of speech. New
York: Academic Press, 1975.

Straight, H.S. Auditory versus articulatory phonological processes and their development in children. In G.H. Yeni-
Komshian, J.F. Kavanagh & C.A. Ferguson (Eds.), Child
phonology: Production (Vol. 1). New York: Academic Press,
1980.

Strange, W., & Broen, P.A. Perception and Production of
approximate consonants by 3 year-olds: A first study. In
G.H. Yeni-Komshian, J.F. Kavanagh & C.A. Ferguson (Eds.),
Child phonology: Perception (Vol. 2). New York: Academic
Press, 1980.

Studdert-Kennedy, M. Speech perception. Language and Speech,
1980, 23, 45-65.

Studdert-Kennedy, M., Liberman, A., Harris, K., & Cooper, F.
Role of formant transitions in the voiced-voiceless distinction for stops. Journal of the Acoustical Society
of America, 1970, 55, 653-659.

Summerfield, Q. Use of visual information for phonetic perception. Phonetica, 1979, 36, 314-331.

Sweitzer, R.S. Audiologic evaluation of the infant and young
child. In B.F. Jaffe (Ed.), Hearing loss in children.
Baltimore: University Park Press, 1977.

Tallal, R., & Stark, R.E. Speech perception of language-
     delayed children. In G.H. Yeni-Komshian, J.F. Kavanagh &
     C.A. Ferguson (Eds.), Child phonology: Perception (Vol.
     2). New York: Academic Press, 1980.

Tallal, P., Stark, R., Kallman, C., & Mellits, D. Perceptual
     constancy for phonemic categories. Applied Psycholin-
     guistics, 1980, 1, 49-64.

Tanaka, Y., & Arayama, T. Fetal responses to acoustic stimu-
     li. Practica Oto-Rhinolaryngologica, 1969, 31, 269-273.

Taylor, D.J., & Mencher, G.T. Neonate response: the effect of
     infant state and auditory stimuli. Archives of Otolar-
     yngology, 1972, 95, 120-124.

Taylor, M.M., & Creelman, C.D. PEST: efficient estimates of
     probability functions. Journal of the Acoustical Society
     of America, 1967, 41, 782-787.

Thompson, G., & Weber, B.A. Responses of infants and young
     children to behavior observation audiometry. Journal of
     Speech and Hearing Disorders, 1974, 39, 140-147.

Thomson, J.R., & Chapman, R.S. Who is 'Daddy' revisited: the
     status of two year olds' over-extended words in use and
     comprehension. Journal of Child Language, 1977, 4, 359-
     375.

Thornton, A., Mendel, M.I., & Anderson, C. Effects of stim-
     ulus frequency and intensity on the middle components of
     the averaged auditory electroencephalic response.
     Journal of Speech and Hearing Research, 1977, 29, 81-94.

Trehub, S.E., Bull, D., & Schneider, B.A. Infants' detection
     of speech in noise. Journal of Speech and Hearing Re-
     search, 1981, 24, 202-206.

Trehub, S.E., Bull, D., & Schneider, B.A. Infant speech and
     nonspeech perception: A review and re-evaluation. In
     R.L. Schiefelbusch & D. Bricker (Eds.), Early language:
     Acquisition and intervention. Baltimore: University
     Park Press, 1981.

Trehub, S.E. Schneider, B.A., & Bull, D. Effect of reinforce-
     ment on infants' performance in an auditory detection
     task. Developmental Psychology, 1981, 17, 872-877.

Trehub, S.E., Schneider, B.A., & Endman, M. Developmental changes in infants' sensitivity to octave-band noises. Journal of Experimental Child Psychology, 1980, 29, 283-293.

Trune, D.R. Influence of neonatal cochlear removal on size and density of cochlear nuclear neurons. Anat. Rec., 1978, 190, 566.

Trune, D.R. Influence of neonatal cochlear removal on the dendritic morphology of cochlear nuclear neurons. Abstracts of the Fourth Midwinter Research Meeting, Association for Research in Otolaryngology, 1981, 65. (Abstract)

Van De Water, T.R. Effects of the statoacoustic ganglion complex upon the growing otocyst. Annals of Otology, Rhinology and Laryngology, Suppl. (33), 1976, 85, 1-32.

Van De Water, T.R., & Ruben, R.J. Organ culture of the mammalian inner ear. Acta Oto-laryngologica, 1971, 71, 303-312.

Van De Water, T.R., & Ruben, R.J. Quantification of the 'in vitro' development of the mouse embryo inner ear. Annals of Otology, Rhinology and Laryngology, 1973, Suppl. 4, 82, 19-21.

Van Riper, C. Speech correction: Principles and methods. Englewood Cliffs, New Jersey: Prentice Hall, 1939.

Vanvik, Arne. The phonetic-phonemic development of a Norwegian child. Norsk Tidsskrift for Sprogvidenskap, XXIV, Oslo, 1971.

Voots, R.J., Harker, L.A., & Mendel, M.I. Three-way ERA system simultaneously collects ECochG, early and middle responses. Journal of the Acoustical Society of America, 1976, 60, S16(A).

Warren, R.M., Obusek, C.J., Farmer, R.M., & Warren, R.P. Auditory sequence: confusion of patterns other than speech or music. Science, 1969, 164, 586-587.

Wedenberg, E. Auditory training of deaf and of hard of hearing children. Acta Oto-laryngologica, 1954, 110, (Suppl.)

Wedenberg, E. Prenatal tests of hearing. Acta Otolaryngo-
    logica, 1965, 206. (Suppl.)

Weir, R.H. Some questions on the child's learing of phonology.
    In F. Smith & G. Miller (Eds.), The genesis of language.
    Cambridge, Mass: M.I.T. Press, 1966.

Whetnall, E. The deaf child. Practitioner, 1955, 174, 375-
    384.

Wiesel, T.N., & Hubel, D.H. Extent of recovery from the
    effects of visual deprivation in kittens. Journal of
    Neurophysiology, 1965, 28, 1060-1972.

Wilson, V.J., & Melvill Jones, G. Mammalian vestibular phys-
    iology. New York: Plenum Press, 1979.

Wilson, W.R. Assessment of auditory abilities in infants. In
    F.D. Minifie & L.L. Lloyd (Eds.), Communicative and Cog-
    nitive abilities: Early behavioral assessment. Balti-
    more: University Park Press, 1978.

Wilson, W.R. Auditory perception. Paper presented at the
    Annual Meeting of the Society for Ear, Nose and Throat
    Advances in Children, Lake Buena Vista, Florida, 1981.

Wilson, W.R., Folsom, R.C., & Widen, J.E. Hearing impairment
    in Down syndrome children. In G.T. Mencher & S.E. Gerber
    (Eds.), The multiply-handicapped hearing-impaired child.
    New York: Grune & Stratton, Inc., in press.

Wilson, W.R., Moore, J.M., & Thompson, G. Auditory thresholds
    of infants utilizing visual reinforcement audiometry
    (VRA). Paper presented at the convention of the American
    Speech and Hearing Association, Houston, 1976.

Wittgenstein, L. Philosophical investigation. New York:
    Macmillan Publishing Co., 1958.

Wolf, K.E., & Goldstein, R. Middle component averaged elec-
    troencephalic responses to tonal stimuli from normal
    neonates. Archives of Otolaryngology, 1978, 104, 508-
    513.

Wolf, K.E., & Goldstein, R. Middle component AERs from neo-
    nates to low-level tonal stimuli. Journal of Speech and
    Hearing Research, 1980, 23, 185-201.

Wood, C. Discriminability, response bias, and phoneme cate-
    gories in discrimination of voice onset time. Journal
    of the Acoustical Society of America, 1976, 60, 1381-
    1389.

Yeni-Komshian, G.H., Kavanagh, J.F., & Ferguson, C.A. Child
    phonology: Perception (Vol. 2). New York: Academic
    Press, 1980.

Yoneshige, Y., & Elliott, L.L. Pure-tone sensitivity and ear
    canal pressure at threshold in Children and Adults.
    Journal of the Acoustical Society of America, 1981, 70,
    1272-1276.

Author Index

Subject Index

Academic achievement
  effect of environmental noise
    on, 183
Acoustic analysis
  in infant babbling, 226, 230
Acoustic events. *See also* Auditory
    stimuli
  behavior of newborns in
    response to, 139, 140, 141,
    142, 143, 144
  discrimination of, 139
  frequency bandwidth in, 140,
    141, 142, 143, 144
  as most effective stimuli for
    infants, 139, 140, 141, 142,
    143, 144
Acoustic response
  of children
    behavioral, 123, 126
    constitution of, 139
    in the fetus, 37, 139
    of infants, 167, 168, 169, 170,
      178, 179, 180, 181
    autonomic, 169
    behavioral, 125, 126, 169, 180
    effect of meaning on, 278
    electrophysiological, 125
    physiological, 169
  of neonates, 139–146
    behavioral, 37
    as defined by the Nova Scotia
      Conference on Early
      Identification of Hearing
      Loss, 140, 141

effect of stimulus complexity
    on, 143
  electrophysiological, 37, 91
  electrophysiological response
    patterns, 91
Acoustic signal
  in the general model of auditory
    perception, 145
  sound integration and
    differentiation, 143, 144
Acoustic stimuli. *See also* Acoustic
    events
  auditory signal, auditory stimuli
    and psychoacoustics, 141
Acoustic trauma
  damage to inner ear, 65, 71, 73,
    74
Acoustics
  and auditory differentiation,
    143, 144
  and auditory discrimination,
    140–143
  and auditory integration, 143,
    144
  and categorization, 141–143
  dimensions of, 140
Adults
  auditory thresholds of, 140, 146,
    174, 175
  categorization in, 272
  cognition in, 245
  formal audiometric testing of, 169
  norms on, as related to children,
    182

a
b
3 c
4 d
5 e
6 f
7 g
8 h
9 i
8 0 j